HOPE

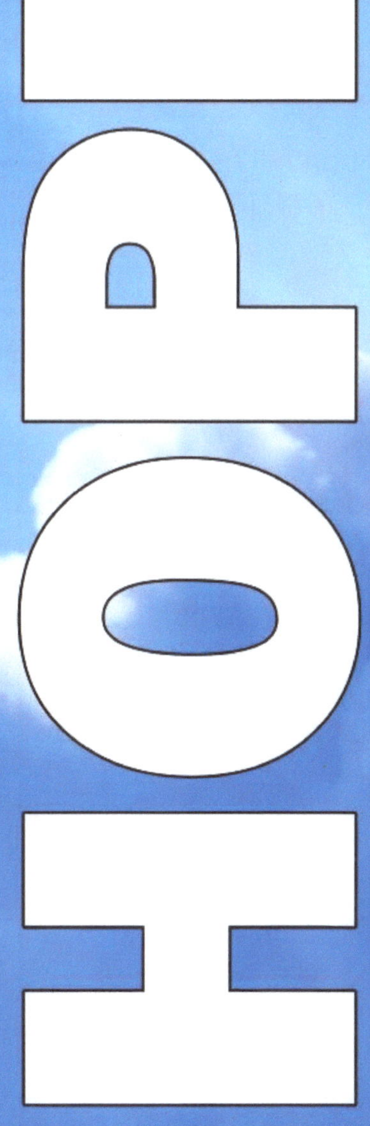

September 2017

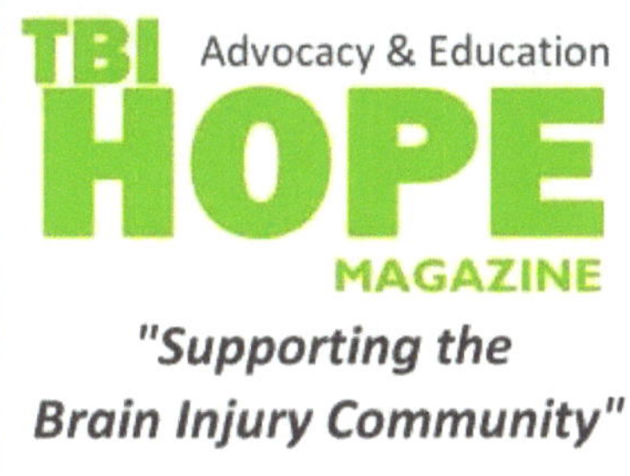

Welcome

TBI HOPE MAGAZINE

Serving All Impacted by Brain Injury

September 2017

Publisher
David A. Grant

Editor
Sarah Grant

Contributing Writers
Karl Heller
Thomas Henson Jr.
Cyndi Kamps
Jim Martin
Sean Montgomery
Norma Myers
Angela Nicholson
Carol Svec
Barbara Webster
Barbara Weekley

Amazing Cartoonist
Patrick Brigham

*FREE subscriptions at
www.TBIHopeMagazine.com*

Welcome to the September 2017 issue of TBI HOPE Magazine!

It's hard to believe that we are now in full-on fall here in New Hampshire. From apple picking to corn mazes, there is no shortage of fun fall activities.

It was seven years ago this month that my wife Sarah and I were enjoying the last fall of the life we used to know. We were only a couple of months away from a brain injury and didn't have a clue what was on the horizon.

So it is for so many others, lives changed in an instant by forces and events outside of their control.

But there is good news! A new and meaningful life can be built after brain injury. Daily, we see, hear from, and watch others within the survivor community who have made life work again. The "new normal" slowly becomes familiar as life takes on new meaning.

We hope you enjoy this early fall issue. Your feedback is always welcome as are your suggestions. We are always trying to improve what we do. You can email me personally at david@tbihopeandinspiration.com.

Peace,

David A. Grant
Publisher

Contents

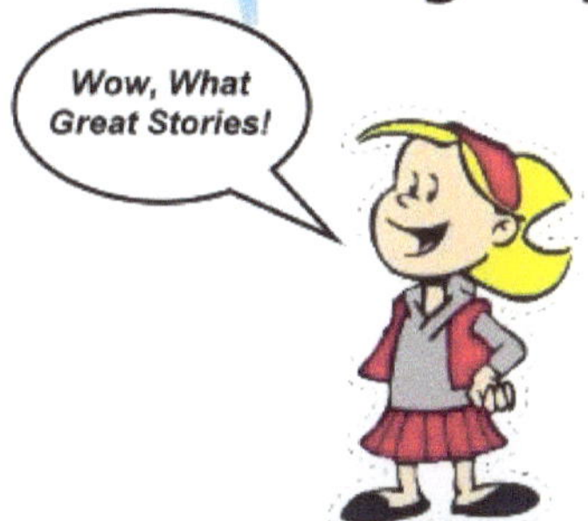

"Bravery is the engine of change."
~Aisha Tyler

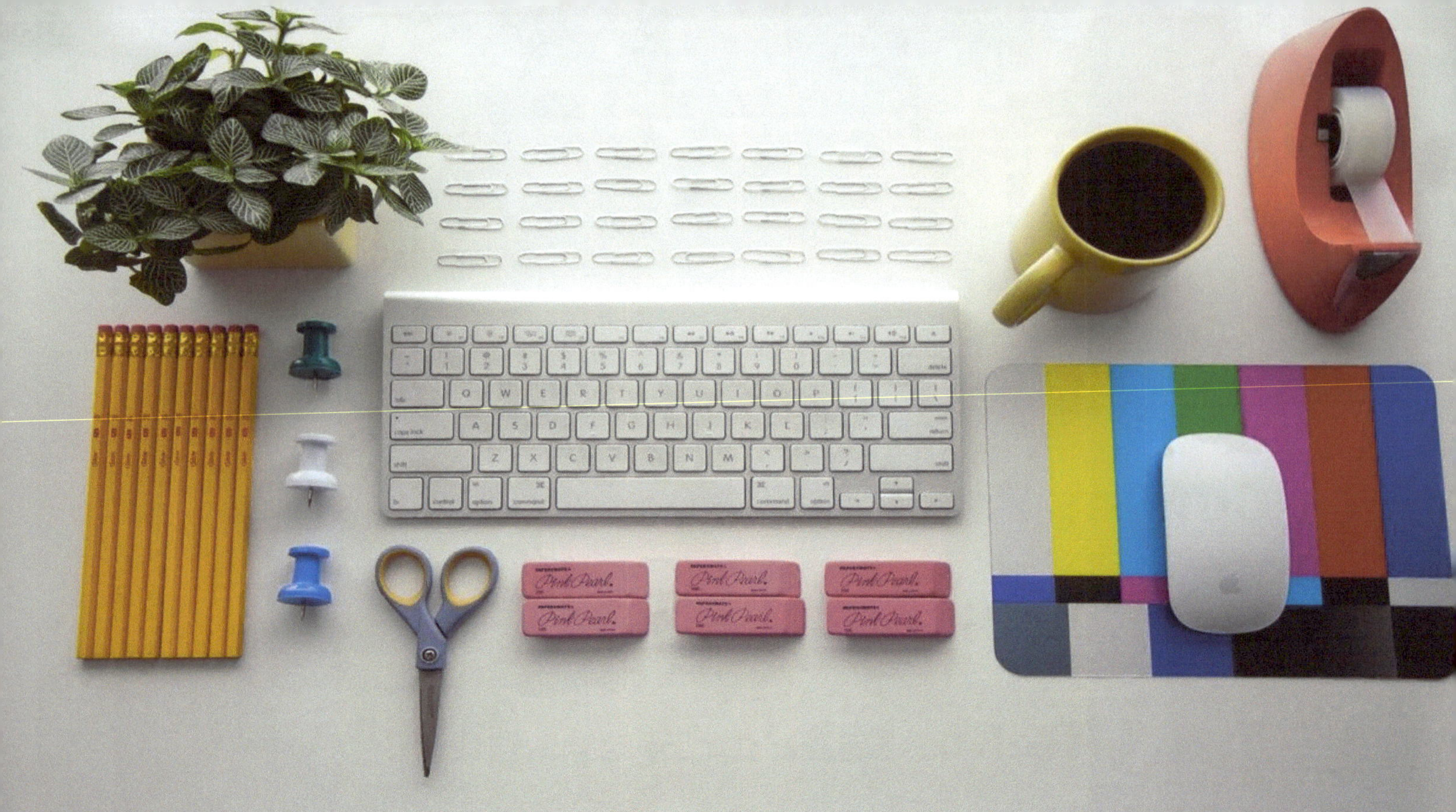

How to Get Organized

By Barbara Webster

You are not alone! Organization and clutter are commonly HUGE problems for brain injury survivors. Why is that? First, keep in mind that your brain is injured and your abilities are compromised. Give yourself a break! Organizing and managing clutter requires making many decisions; the more decisions involved in a task, the harder it is. Second, consider that you have been injured and "out of commission" for a while, maybe a long while, causing a backlog, probably a huge backlog!

So when you can think about tackling your pile of "to do's," just looking at them can overwhelm you, making you feel like you want to run away or just sweep everything into the trash!

Take heart! Below are some helpful suggestions from a recent brainstorming session of the "Amazing" Brain Injury Survivor Support Group in Framingham, MA.

> **Keep in mind that your brain is injured and your abilities are compromised.**

Use a weekly planner or calendar to plan your time and energy and prevent fatigue:

• Refer to it every day - every morning and every evening.
• Take it where ever you go.
• Establish regular times to update and plan ahead.

Set yourself up to succeed:

• Before you begin, prepare a small reward for every small task accomplished!
• Plan to do "hard stuff" and "must do's" at the time of day when your brain is at its best.
• Get your tea/coffee before you start, put on some white noise or soothing music, mute phone alerts and put phones out of sight so that nothing distracts you.
• Work in a clear space, so you won't be distracted. Go to the library if helpful.
• Use planning worksheets.

Paperwork:

• Divide paperwork up into categories. Use different colored folders for each category.
• Establish priorities and start with the "must do's."
• Start small. One issue - one pile - one folder at a time.
• Sometimes you just have to begin; take care of one little thing, to get started.
• Use timers to help you pace yourself and take a break when you start to get signs that you are getting tired.
• If taking a break doesn't help, quit for the day.
• Some days just won't be "good brain days" for complicated paperwork or dealing with clutter.

Clutter:

• PREVENT as much clutter as you can, ELIMINATE the task if you can, DELEGATE if it feels too hard at this time, then BREAK THE TASK DOWN INTO SMALLER STEPS - and get started!
• Touch things once and deal with it then if you can.
• Eliminate junk mail right away; keep a wastebasket close to where you sort the mail.
• Stop magazine subscriptions that are piling up unread.
• Paying bills by phone or online can be helpful.

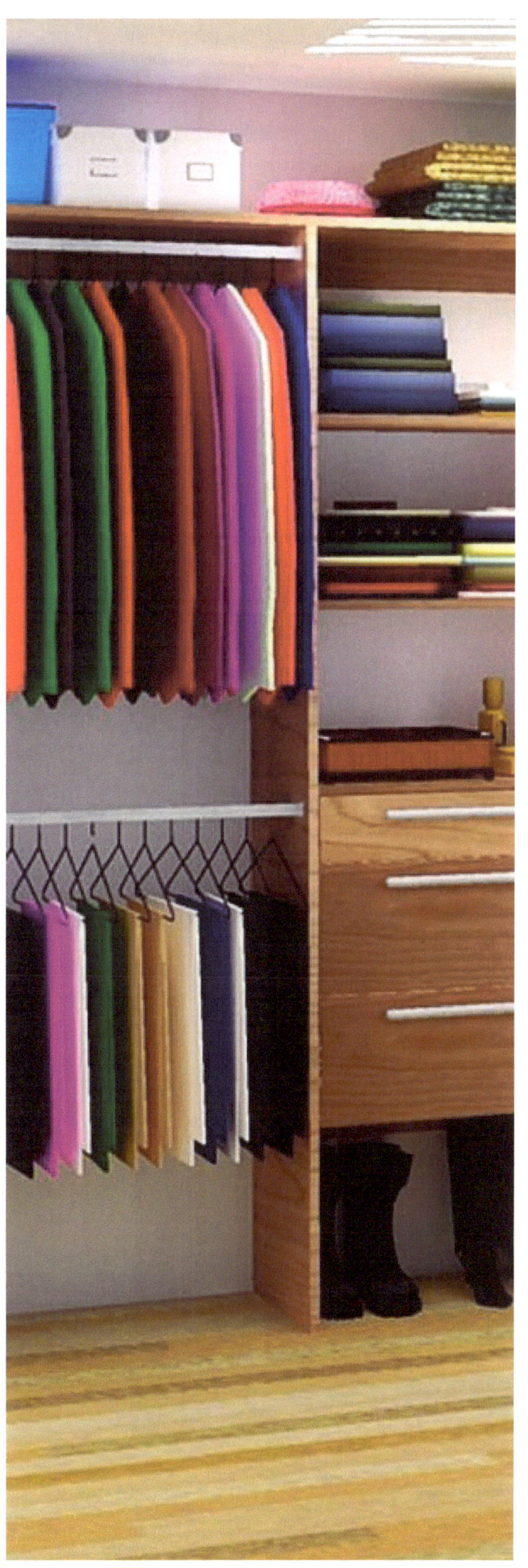

- Start small; one pile - one drawer - one corner at a time.
- Commit to the project: PLAN an hour each day or all the time you have for the next two weeks, until you are caught up.
- Find a "clutter buddy" to work with, or just to check in with and help motivate you.
- Reward any progress! Pat yourself on the back! Do a victory dance! Celebrate by doing something that makes you smile!
- Once you are caught up, plan to spend time each day/week to keep up, so it doesn't get overwhelming again.
- Conquering clutter creates space, in your life and your brain!
- Now, get started!

One other note: it is often necessary, not just nice or helpful but necessary, to enlist some help to help you dig out, catch up and get back on track.

Meet Barbara Webster

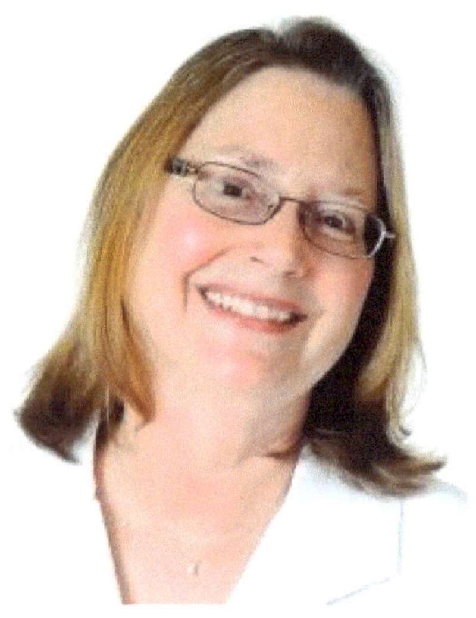

Barbara J. Webster is author of Lost and Found, A Survivors Guide for Reconstructing Life after a Brain Injury, Lash & Assoc. Publishing and a contributor to Chicken Soup for the Traumatic Brain Injury Survivor's Soul.

Barbara has the privilege of facilitating the Brain Injury Survivor Support Group in Framingham since 1995 and works part-time for the Brain Injury Association of Massachusetts assisting other support groups. "I get to do something that I am passionate about and I get to work with good people," Barbara shares.

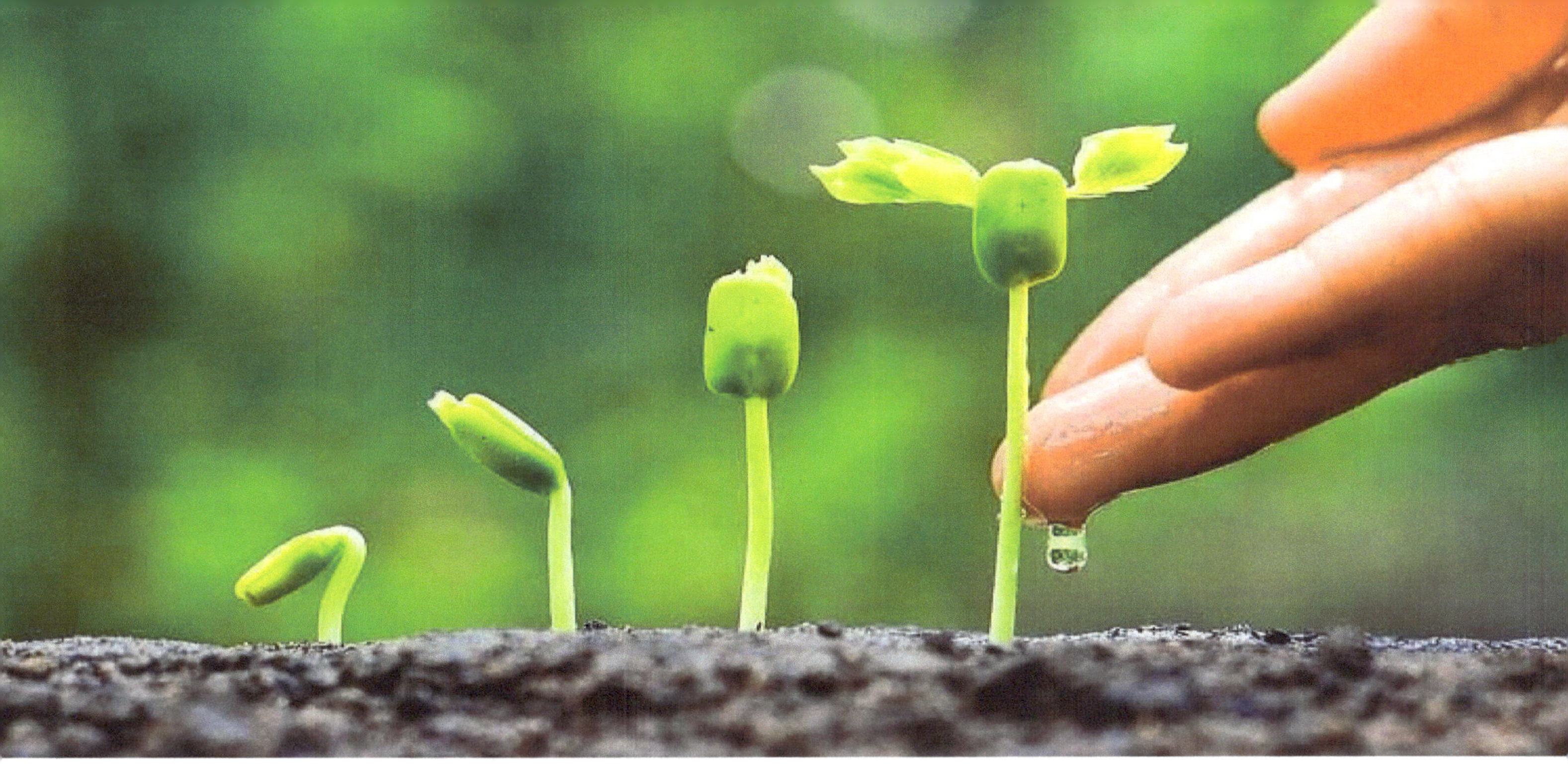

Coming Back to Life

By Karl Heller

It was a beautiful summer day eleven years ago in August of 2006 when everything suddenly changed for me.

Just a few months short of my fiftieth birthday, I was living a gifted life. I had been an accomplished student (third in my high school class), a talented athlete (set records in track), and a sax player selected to my city's district band. I received full scholarship offers from colleges for each of these three skills, and I chose to go to West Point from which I graduated in 1978. After Army active duty service, I joined the working public and eventually found myself moved up to VP of sales for a local Dallas company. Yes, everything was going very nicely for me. I mention all of the above, not to try to impress you with how accomplished I may think I am, but only to point out how quickly things can change if you were to lose it all.

> **In an instant, a motor vehicle accident very nearly killed me, and I found out how dramatically things can change.**

In an instant, a motor vehicle accident very nearly killed me, and I found out how dramatically things can change. I was on the way to a Rangers baseball game when I ran into stopped traffic for an accident that had happened in front of me on the freeway. While I was waiting to move past the stoppage, a driver behind me fell asleep in his car, while moving at full speed. He damaged ten vehicles but managed to hit me first. Fortunately for me, emergency personnel were already on-hand for the accident in front of me, and they were able to get to me quickly. They wrangled me out of my totaled vehicle, and after restarting my heart sent me by helicopter to the emergency room. The initial prognosis was not good.

Every rib in my body was broken in at least one place; both lungs were punctured, numerous organs were damaged, and in general, it was estimated that I had a low chance to survive (2 out of 15). After two weeks in intensive care attached to God-knows-what-all to save my life, I was well enough to spend the next three months in bed at the

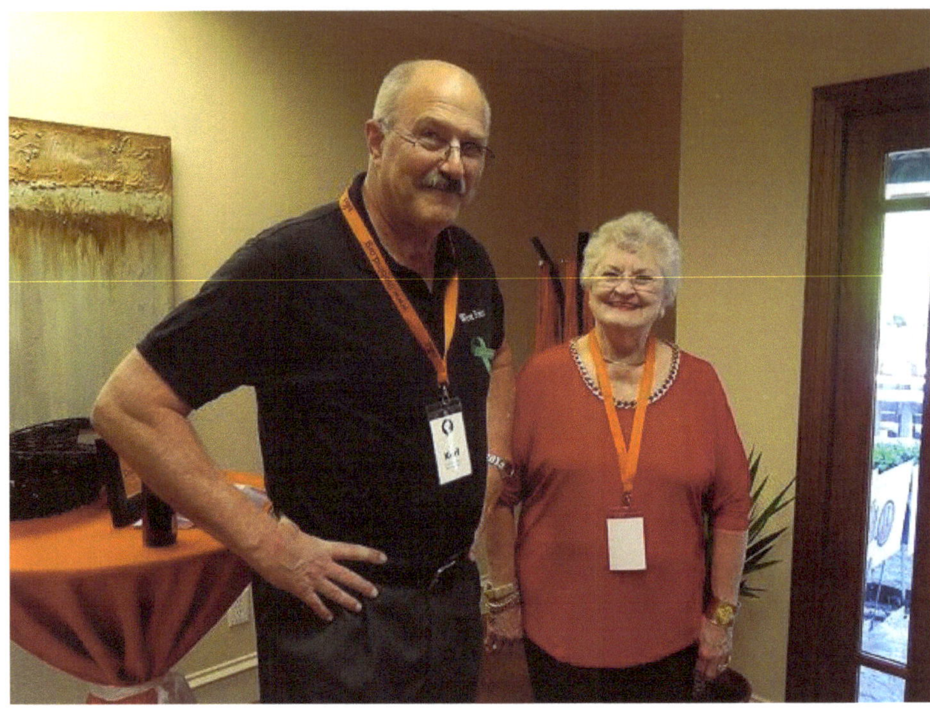

hospital. Then began the real hard part: therapy for the brain injury that I had sustained during my accident.

My losses were significant and numerous. I couldn't walk and used a wheelchair to move around. My entire right side was initially paralyzed, and as I healed, there were constant challenges with raising my right arm and moving my right leg.

> **The worst, however, was the discovery that I had completely lost my communication skills.**

The worst, however, was the discovery that I had completely lost my communication skills. I couldn't read, and upon testing was found to be able to identify only two of the 26 letters of the alphabet. Needless to say, I couldn't write anything because I couldn't recognize and spell the words out. I couldn't speak in a coherent fashion. Initially, I used one noun to describe everything: "noodle."

In my head, I was saying everything that I was thinking, but I could tell from the reaction of those who were listening to me that something was desperately wrong. "Noodle" this and "noodle" that was not getting the job done. As is blatantly obvious, the new me is very different from the old me described earlier.

After nearly two-and-a-half years of therapy and a lot of hard work by the therapists, I came back to life. I am now able to read at a post-college level. I can write to nearly the same degree. I am speaking beyond "noodle" now, and find many opportunities to talk to the general public about brain injury subjects. On the physical side, I have completed several 5K road races, and although my right leg still wants to drag a bit, I am planning to achieve longer runs.

In all, I am very thankful that my accident happened while I was heading to meet customers for the game-night out. Considered a business accident, I was fully covered by insurance to help with my recovery through the full two-and-a-half years that I continued to progress. Not a fraction of the brain injury patients that I met along the way were as fortunate as I was.

I was lucky to have had such support. The lesson learned is that recovery from a brain injury is most likely one of the hardest things that a person is ever going to experience. It takes hard work, persistence, a positive attitude, and help from people who know what you need to do to recover. The good news is that you can recover, and the better news is that the worst day of your brain injury was the first day. Everything gets better if you put in the effort. It is all up to you to continue working.

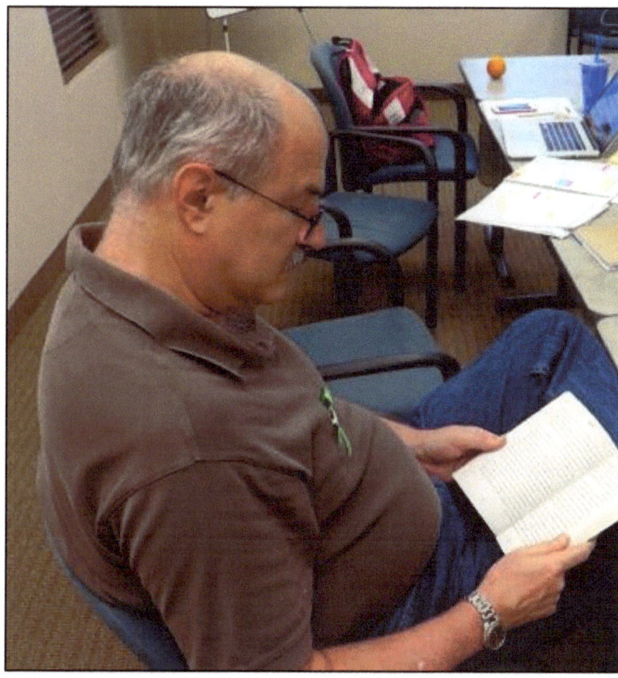

Meet Karl Heller

Karl Heller is an Ex-Officio Member of the Board of Directors, BIND: Brain Injury Network of Dallas. Prior to Karl's traumatic brain injury in 2006, he worked as the Vice President of Sales for Southwestern Battery Supply in Garland, Texas.

Karl earned a Bachelor's degree in Engineering from the US Military Academy at West Point and an MBA from Oklahoma City University. Karl served for six years in the Army. He enjoys a good steak, cheering for the Dallas Stars and the Texas Rangers. Karl joined the BIND Board of Directors three years ago and also participates in the program as a team leader for the Wellness Unit.

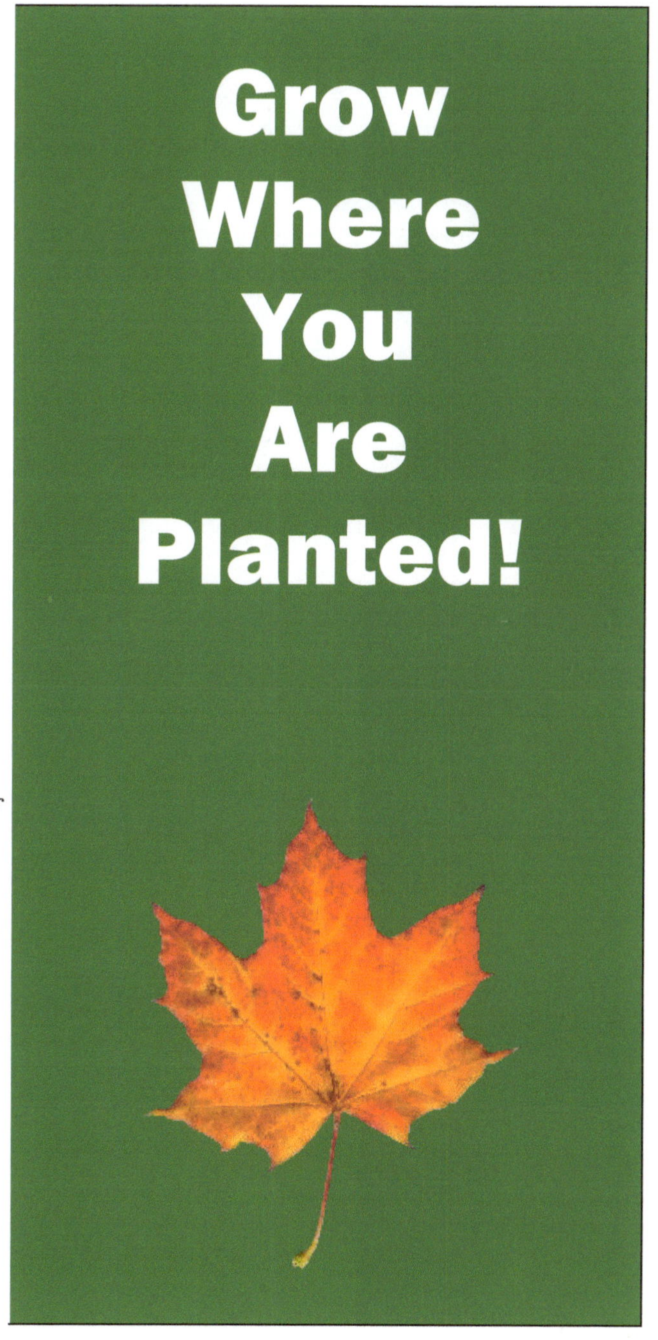

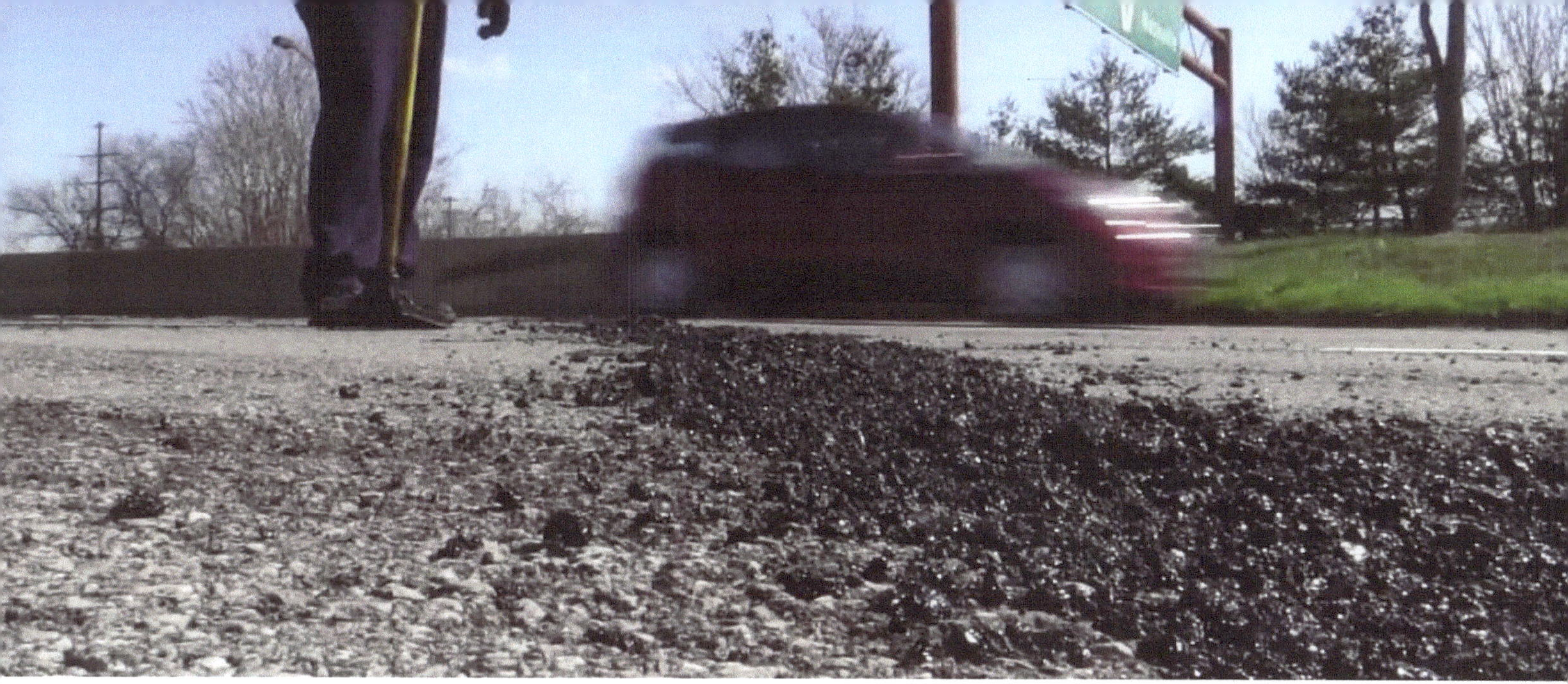

Our New Normal

By Cyndi Kamps

On February 8, 2011, our normal world was turned upside down when Bob was hit by a car. He sustained a critical and severe closed head injury resulting in a diffuse axonal injury (DAI), and our new normal began. It took only a moment to change our world into a nightmare. This nightmare brought pain, heartache, and constant drama to everyday life.

My husband Bob was fifty years old when he suffered a severe closed head injury at the hands of an incompetent driver. As a crew member for the Michigan Department of Transportation (MDOT), Bob routinely shoveled tar into the many pot holes on Michigan's weather-beaten roads. It was a Tuesday evening at 6:30 pm when the driver of an SUV slammed into two of the MDOT crew members resulting in Bob's life changing and horrific injury (the second crew member sustained minor injuries).

There were many things in Bob's favor when the injury occurred. He was just one mile away from a level one trauma center, he didn't break any major bones, and his spinal cord was unharmed. And, he was "young-ish" (the trauma doctor's words). His journey over the next seven months brought him to four different institutions with many tragic, triumphant, and tumultuous days.

> **There were many things in Bob's favor when the injury occurred.**

Bob spent five weeks in the critical care unit at a level one trauma center, where he was hooked up to all kinds of gadgets to keep him alive. He was kept in a medically induced coma for a few weeks to allow his brain to heal. As they slowly began to reduce the

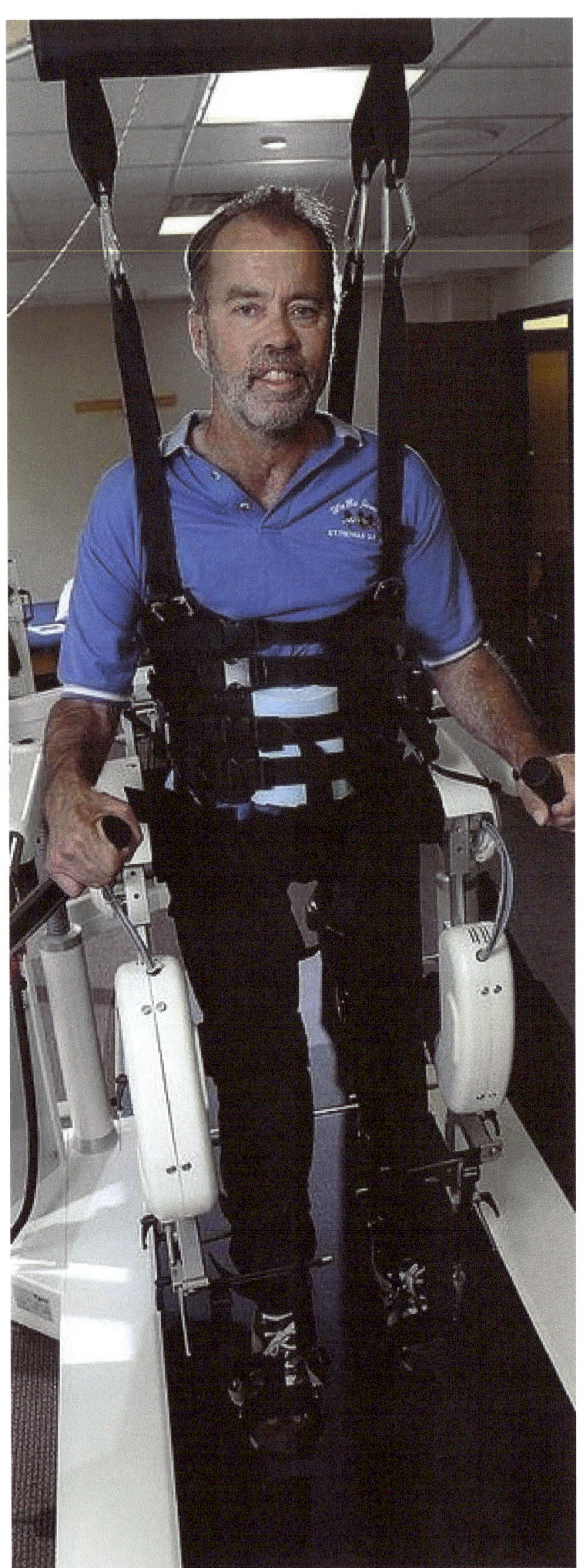

amount of the drugs, they were hoping for Bob to regain consciousness and to interact with his environment. Unfortunately, he didn't progress as they had hoped.

We had a conundrum: his condition wasn't serious enough to keep him in critical care, but he wasn't well enough to move to a regular hospital unit.

After gathering information and talking to the medical staff, we decided to move Bob to a long term acute care hospital (L-TAC). Bob spent ten days at the L-TAC where he continued to receive focused care. He also started therapy by receiving passive exercises where the therapists moved Bob's arms and legs for him. The therapists also positioned him to sit on the side of the bed. It took two therapists and about ten minutes to get him to this position. It was thrilling, exhilarating, heartbreaking and tremendous to see him making progress. Heartbreaking because he had to go through it, but so incredibly exciting because he was making progress.

After ten days at the L-TAC, Bob improved enough to move to a sub-acute rehabilitation center where he spent three months gaining strength, relearning to eat, walk, talk, and use his arms. He entered this facility requiring full care, including the use of lift equipment, called a "Hoyer," to get him in and out of bed, a tracheotomy for help with breathing, and the use of a feeding tube. At the end of the three months, Bob was able to transfer from his bed to his chair with just one person helping. He stood on his own two feet with no balance issues, his tracheotomy was gone, and he could eat and drink regular food – no restrictions. He did still have his feeding tube, but that was just in case of emergency (which never happened, thank goodness).

The last inpatient institution for Bob was the acute care rehabilitation hospital where he spent two more months with more intensive therapy, and they finally were able to remove the feeding tube. His therapy sessions consisted of physical, occupational, speech, and recreational therapies each for thirty minutes, twice a day. That's four hours of intense therapy.

Thankfully, they split that up throughout the day and built in rest periods so his brain could have a break and he could remain successful in the therapies.

So, if you're keeping track, that's five weeks in critical care, ten days in L-TAC, three months in the sub-acute rehab hospital, and two months in the acute care rehab hospital. That brings us to the end of August 2011 when Bob finally got to come home. It was one of the most exciting and terrifying days of my life. He no longer required professional medical/therapeutic treatments as an inpatient but still needed 24/7 supervision. After being near death, was he really ready to come home? I was petrified and over-the-moon all at the same time.

For the next three years, Bob continued physical, occupational, speech, and recreational therapy as an outpatient. He learned how to perform "activities of daily living (ADLs)" by adapting and utilizing tools that supported his limitations. Again, Bob had many things in his favor. The injury affected his right side. Thankfully, he's left handed! (Try brushing your teeth with your non-dominant hand. If you're right handed, brush with your left. Impossible.) His speech is clear but soft, which has improved and continues to improve to this day. He has mild aphasia, which typically happens when he's overly tired or agitated. And, as I mentioned earlier, he didn't have any other serious injuries. It was just all in his head.

So, Bob spent over four years in structured therapy. He officially graduated in June of 2014. He continues a daily exercise routine at home, and he can walk when holding on to a railing. We don't like to focus on what he can't do but rather what he can. He has physical limitations on his right side requiring a wheelchair to get around. His brain injury requires that he have 24/7 supervision for the rest of his life. A diffuse axonal brain injury is similar to shaken baby syndrome. There is damage all throughout the brain making it very difficult for medical professionals to predict an outcome. This unpredictability worked in our favor because we had no expectations and any progress Bob made was and continues to be truly miraculous. Despite all that he's been through, Bob continues to be a positive, uplifting, and happy man. It is truly a blessing and a joy to have him with us. We continue to be thankful and feel very blessed with the support from family, friends, co-workers, and people we haven't even met.

Meet the Kamps

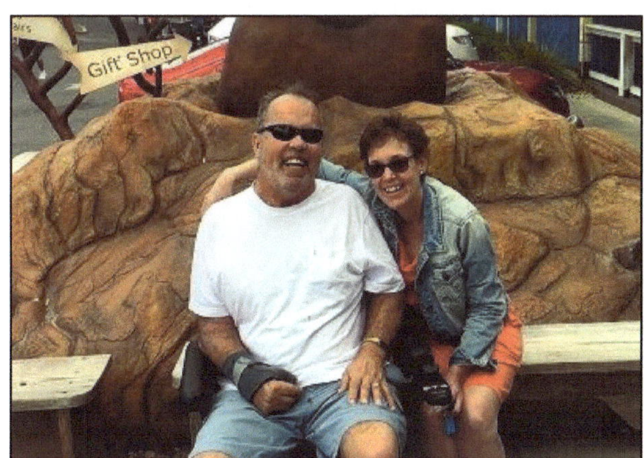

Bob and Cyndi Kamps grew up in Western Michigan and currently reside in the Grand Rapids area. Bob's severe traumatic brain injury brought setbacks, highs and lows and many tears. However, his wife Cyndi never wavered from her devotion, courage, strength and love, a love which, along with a superb team of professionals, brought Bob through the worst of times and helped him regain hope and freedom. They enjoy golfing together using Bob's adaptive golf equipment, vacationing in Florida and a cup of good coffee.

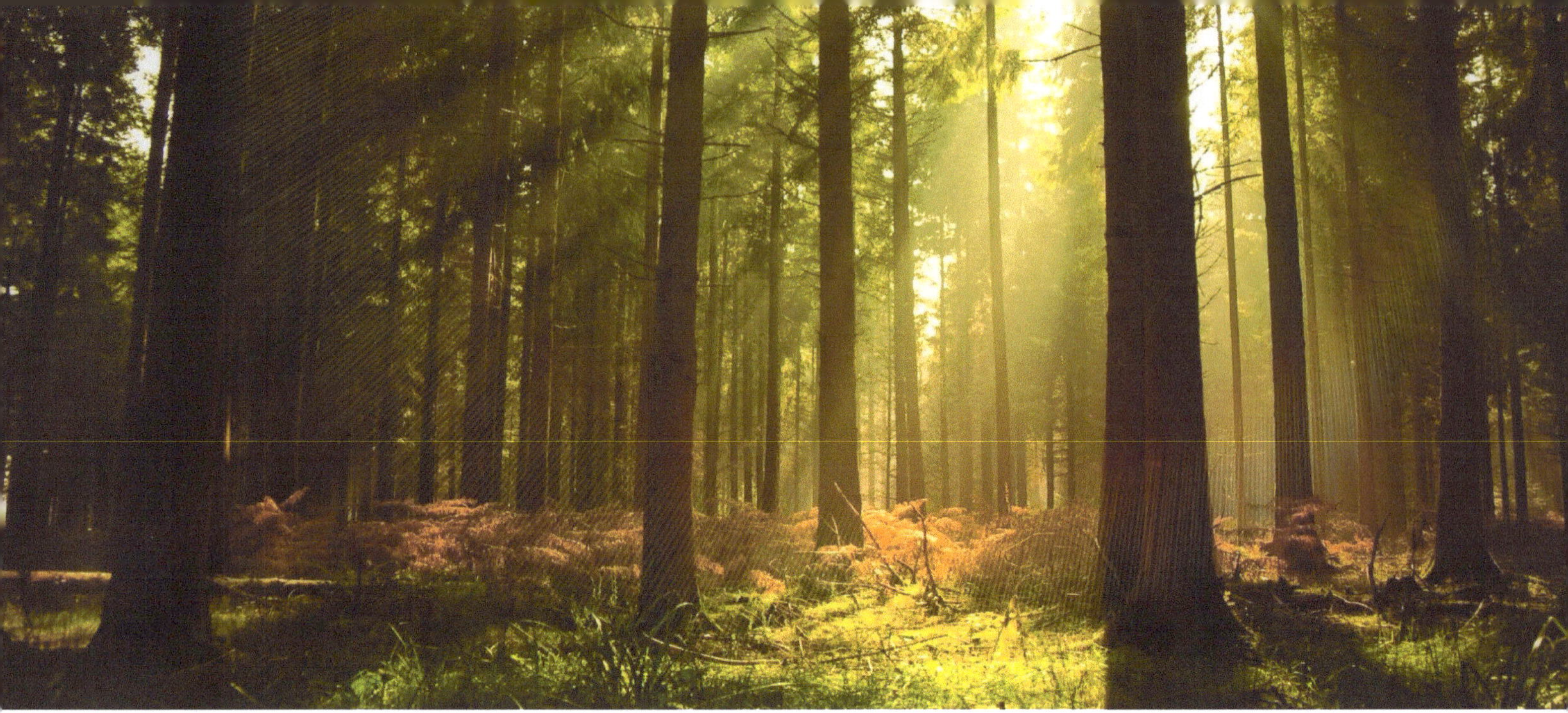

Two Life-Sustaining Questions

By Norma Myers

All parents are faced with the same common questions while raising their children. We were no different. *Will we be good parents? Will our boys be healthy? How will they do in school? What professions will they choose? Will they meet their soulmates and make us grandparents?* These are normal, casual, and expected questions until your worst nightmare becomes a reality. For us, the nightmare was a fatal car accident that took our firstborn son and left our only surviving son with a severe Traumatic Brain Injury (TBI) and a life without his brother, his best friend.

When we answered a knock on our door in the early hours of the morning expecting to see our sons, we were instead looking into the bleak faces of police officers as questions immediately started formulating. Because of the protective layer of shock that consumed my body, I couldn't audibly ask the searing questions that I so desperately needed to be answered: *What caused the accident? Did my boys suffer? How long did they wait for help*? The agonizing questions kept swirling in my head, spinning like a washing machine stuck on the spin cycle.

The once casual questions of early parenthood turned into heart-wrenching screams, assaulting my heart like a machine gun stuck in an automatic mode. Unfortunately, some of my questions were answered without being voiced: *Aaron wouldn't get to experience the magical moment of saying, "I do!" He was robbed of the joys of fatherhood. No more hunting trips with his buddies. No more quality time with his brother. Family beach vacations for the four of us are now memories from the past.*

In the blink of an eye for our sons, and with an unwelcome knock on our door for my husband and me, our family changed in a way that we could not even begin to comprehend. While we didn't physically change addresses, it felt as if we had morphed into a new life full of unknowns. The chapter of our life as an intact family of four was removed from our parental handbook; in return, hospital staff offered a manual about TBI, and the funeral home handed us a brochure addressing grieving the loss of a child. These resources were meant to be a comfort, but all I wanted to do was find a shredder and do to those resources exactly what the accident did to me, tear them into a million pieces, with no chance of being put back together in the same way again.

The merry-go-round of questions left me feeling queasy from the never-ending thoughts of what's next. The questions changed with each season of recovery coupled with each season of grief; *will Steven survive and what will recovery look like? How will I plan a life celebration for Aaron? How do I go about securing resources for Steven's rehabilitation and recovery? How does a family recover from such a catastrophic loss? When will we grieve? Will our marriage survive the greatest test of our thirty-two years together? Will our family, friends, and community continue to be there for us?*

As we watched our surviving son fight his way back to us, the recovery road wasn't easy. There were insurance battles. There were tears when therapists gave up too easily. And then there was our favorite: reminding healthcare providers that Steven could answer their questions himself, and on top of that, they didn't have to yell—his TBI didn't cause deafness. If I sound a bit sarcastic, it's because TBI has forced us to encounter the

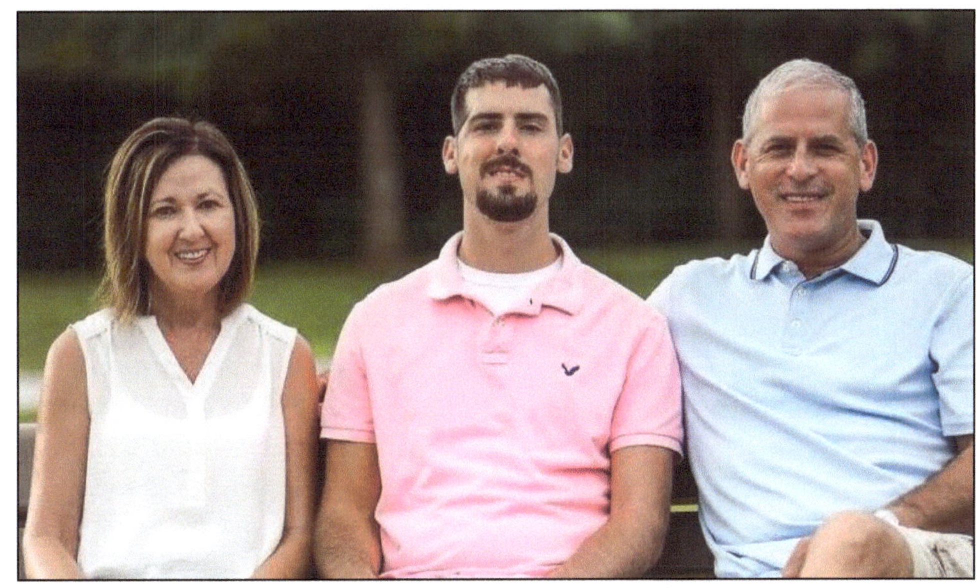

worst of the worst coupled with the best of the best. There are defeats that lead to tears and celebrations that are never taken for granted.

TBI alone causes a unique kind of grief, but when it collides with devastation from the death of your other child, it causes guilt for smiling. Laughter is followed by tears, not the kind of welcomed tears from a belly laugh, but tears from the remnants of a broken heart and ultimately experiencing a sense of sadness every single day, even when feeling happy. It's a complex journey.

I remember in the early days following the accident. Amid the chaos, and despite the unknowns, my husband and I joined hands and hearts asking God to give us the physical and emotional strength to make whatever sacrifices necessary to ensure that we were by Steven's side providing security and support, all while doing everything humanly possible to keep Aaron's memory alive.

As we approach five years since the knock on our door, we are thankful that Steven doesn't let his TBI define him. We proudly watch as he sets, pursues, and achieves goals. TBI is an invisible disability; it can be very lonely if people are unwilling to get out of their comfort zone, become educated, and just show up. We are thankful for those that see beyond Steven's TBI and have the privilege of being exposed to his positive outlook on life. He possesses a *never-give-up* attitude and an infectious smile that reminds me of his brother.

Each day my heart experiences a tidal wave of emotions that threaten to sweep me off my feet. By the grace of God, I stay grounded, always asking myself two life-sustaining questions:

What would Aaron want me to do? What does Steven need?

I choose to believe that Steven needs and deserves the same mom he and his brother have always known, a mom who offers unconditional love, puts family first, forgives freely and never gives up. I know this is what Aaron would want.

Life goes on with traumatic brain injuries, with the loss of loved ones, with broken hearts, and unanswered questions. I am committed to remaining by Steven's side as he continues healing both physically and emotionally, and I will speak Aaron's name daily to keep his memory alive. I will continue to travel this path that was paved for me with grace and faith, trusting in strength that comes from God who so graciously restores my depleted strength daily.

Meet Norma Myers

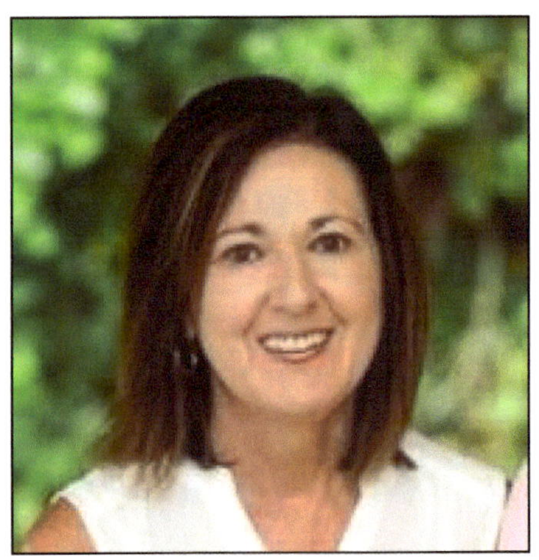

Norma and her husband Carlan spend much of their time supporting their son Steven as he continues on his road to recovery. Norma is an advocate for those recovering from traumatic brain injury.

Her written work has been featured on Brainline.org, a multi-media website that serves the brain injury community. Her family continues to heal.

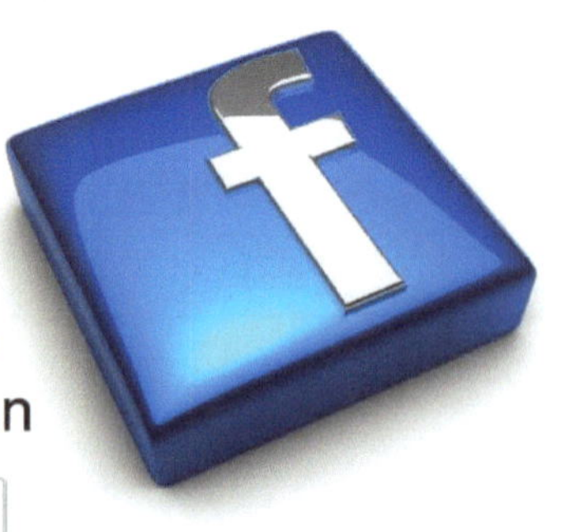

AFTER A TBI, THE DAILY CHALLENGE IS TO LIVE YOUR LIFE FULLY EVERY DAY.

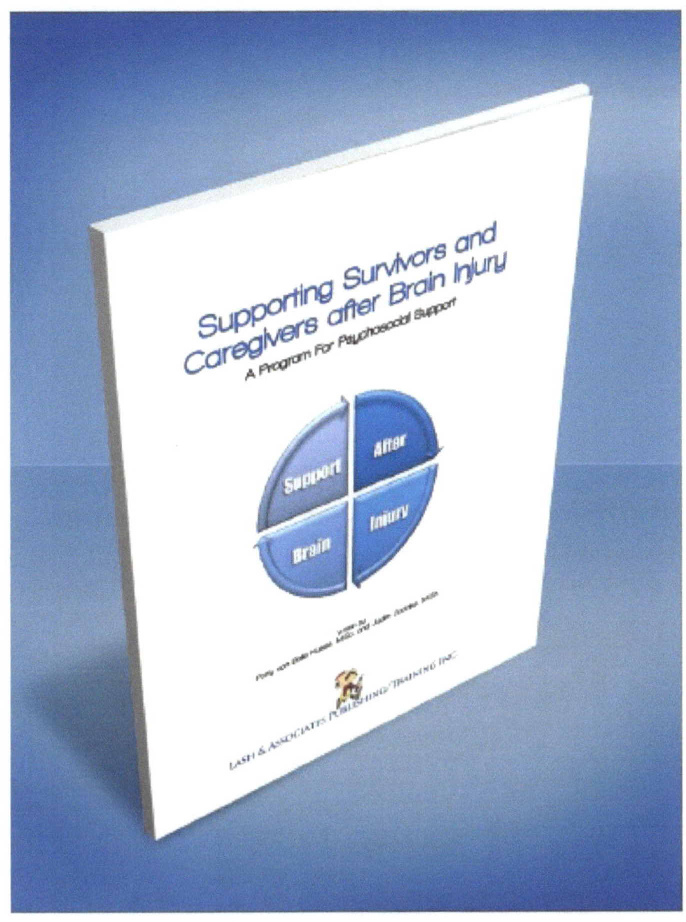

Supporting Survivors and Caregivers after Brain Injury:
A program for psychosocial support

Manual helps develop skills, activities and other tools that promote the survivor regaining control over their life. Supports the survivior living at home, residential program, nursing home, or assisted living facility. Provides insight into changes that the brain has experienced, changes in social networks, perspective change, looking at life in a new way, and maximizing the survivor's quality of life.

LASH & ASSOCIATES PUBLISHING/TRAINING INC.

919-556-0300   www.lapublishing.com

Item: SABI

Sale Price: $24.00

(Reg. $35.00 - Save 31%)

Order now and save!

For details, or to order, go to: https://www.lapublishing.com/brain-injury-recovery/

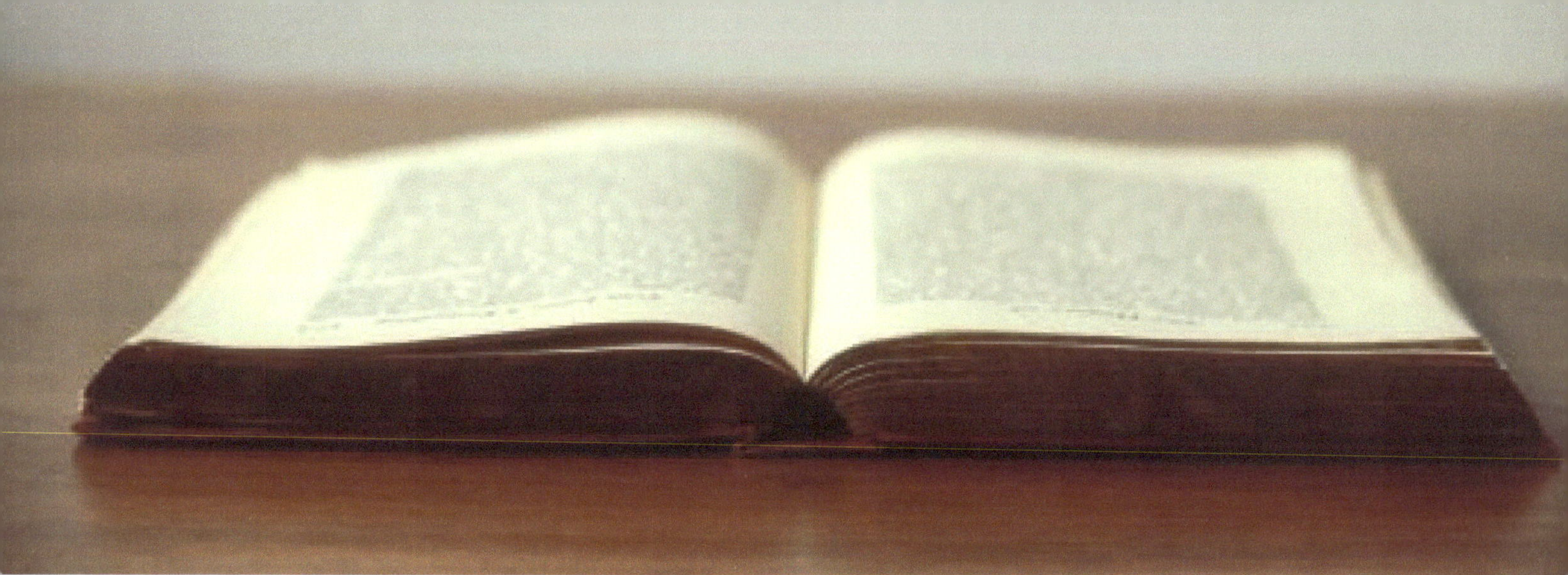

Acceptance is the Answer

By Jim Martin

Following my brain injury, I became challenged with an affinity for alcohol as a means to soothe my emotional state. Fortunately, I'd like to think that I am now in solid recovery, so long as I maintain a healthy balance in life. Balance, much like hope, is not a concept easily defined in mere words. Rather, it has become and hopefully will continue to evolve on a daily basis. I say that from several perspectives: health, physical activity, connection to others, opportunities to volunteer, and perhaps most importantly, finding time to rest and accept that, having experienced a TBI and the resulting memory impairment, I can still be useful and productive to others.

My excessive use of alcohol was a combination of a desire to control my external surroundings, business or otherwise, and a huge dose of self-pity, especially following the TBI accident, hospitalizations, and foster care home experiences I encountered. Despite those experiences, I nonetheless retained hope that the situation would improve. I am fortunate that it has.

> I nonetheless retained hope that the situation would improve. I am fortunate that it has.

That doesn't mean that I'm not desiring to return to my profession of thirty years, jealous of colleagues who are continuing to be successful, and as I age not being able to enjoy many of the physical activities of youth. This is my new reality. Once I became accepting of it, my perspective on life changed. I now continue to seek a balance, or a sense of contentment, that I previously failed to recognize.

Drawing from a passage from a book famous for helping alcoholics, the following has created a new meaning for me in many, many contexts:

"Acceptance is the answer to all my problems today. When I am disturbed, it is because I find some person, place, thing or situation — some fact of my life — unacceptable to me, and I can find no serenity until I accept that person, place, thing, or situation as being exactly the way it is supposed to be at this moment. Nothing, absolutely nothing, happens in God's world by mistake. I need to concentrate not so much on what needs to be changed in the world as on what needs to be changed in me and in my attitudes."

Although the above is drawn from a book primarily devoted to alcoholism, the heartfelt message is the same, whether it be a disease or, in my case, the combination of disease and traumatic brain injury.

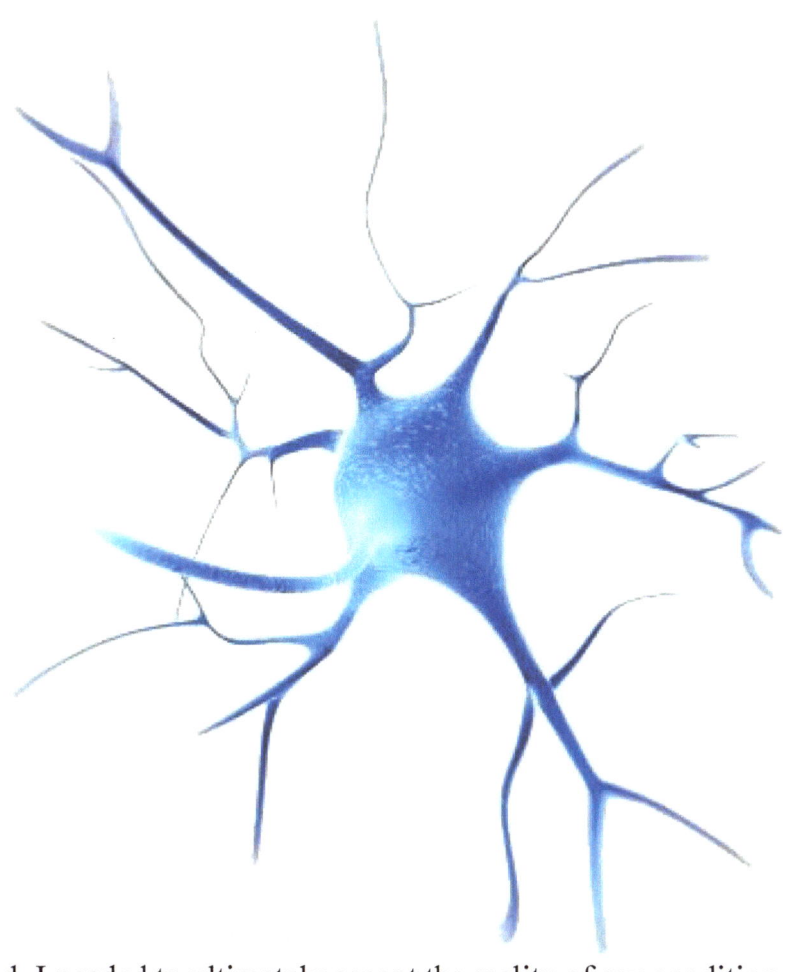

That being said, I have also become more cognizant of how invisible these impairments truly exist. In contrast with the multiple orthopedic and neurological surgeries I've experienced, there has been external evidence of my injury/disability.

The more I struggled to accept my memory impairment and resulting consequences, as well as the effects of my excessive use of alcohol, those were, to most of the world, invisible, especially as I recovered. Initially, I became frustrated with responding to inquiries such as "What do you expect when you're sixtyish" or "What's going to be different now?"

Although I was not capable of responding to such questions because the true answers needed to emanate from my heart, not my head, I needed to ultimately accept the reality of my condition and recognize that I could remain a productive, useful person, unashamed of my impairments, and move forward.

As I continue this new journey, I look forward, and therefore hope, to share my experience in ways which may be helpful to others similarly situated. These efforts have included my participation with the Alzheimer's Association, telling my story at an annual fund raising event entitled Reason to Hope, to medical students from Oregon Health Science University (OHSU), being a liaison to Congressman Earl Blumenauer's Portland office, and connecting with local physicians who treat patients with all forms of memory impairment.

Although my current life is dramatically different than it once was, I am finding productive and enjoyable endeavors to define my existence more fully. So, what's next? I am not sure. I do find hope in being able to communicate with others in similar situations, conveying hope, and seeking solutions. Hope is born while facing the unknown and discovering that one is not alone.

Meet Jim Martin

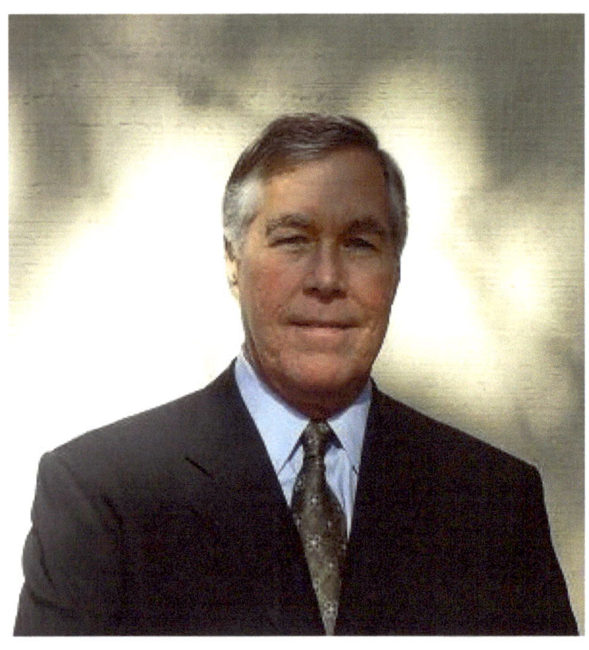

After 30 years practicing law as a trial attorney primarily representing physicians in medical malpractice litigation, Jim is a brain injury survivor whose career ended in December, 2010 when he experienced a significant traumatic brain injury, and resulting permanent memory impairment.

Following an extended period of time learning to accept his new reality, he now volunteers with the Alzheimer's Association, where he is a Board member, attends support group meetings with Brain Injury Connections NW, is a member of Brain Injury Alliance of Oregon, and volunteers at a local Portland, Oregon hospital.

To stay connected with the legal community, Jim mentors newly admitted lawyers with the Oregon State Bar.

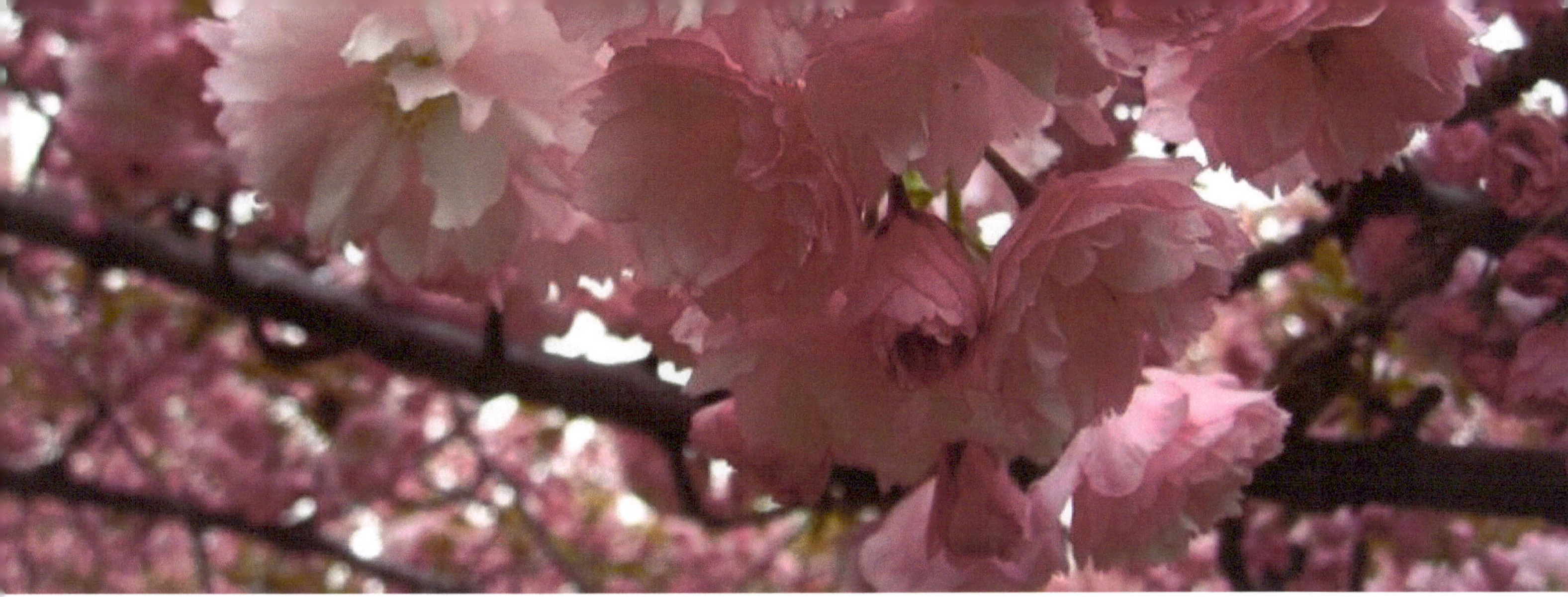

June Never Came
By Barbara Weekley

I thought I had it all worked out in my head. My nine-year caregiving of my mom ended with her death in 2008, and our three sons were grown and living their own lives, so my responsibilities were lessening at home. Pre-accident, Charlie still had a few more years before retirement, so we decided it was time for us! It was all figured out! In June of 2009, I would go on the road with him and experience first-hand many of the places he had told me about over our then almost thirty-three-year marriage.

In May 2009, Charlie was on his way home to me, when the unthinkable happened. Because of a catastrophic highway moment, my husband would spend most of the summer of 2009 in a coma battling multiple injuries and blood loss - including something called a TBI, (which I had never heard of before). For us, June never arrived. By that August, when he began to awaken, I realized the wreck had completely removed the words "we" and "us" from our marriage vocabulary. I was alone and overwhelmed.

> It has been eight years now since the doctors told me he would not survive.

It has been eight years now since the doctors told me he would not survive. But he did! I had to learn how to "compartmentalize" my husband into pre-accident and post-accident people so I could handle things better. Although the dynamic of what made Charlie and me "us" has been altered, we still maintain a kind of oneness without the lovely, intimate bond of whispers in the night. He is high functioning today, yet we still are reminded how different our roles are now. Everything from making a simple decision to emotional and psychological maturity levels have been compromised because of the crash.

Taking care of my husband has been a tremendous learning experience. I had to develop layers of impenetrable skin, and acquire more patience if we were going to survive not only as a couple but as individuals. I learned that I am a strong woman, even though I continue at times to cry in the shower or my car, where Charlie cannot see. I have learned that making decisions for both of us is challenging and that doctors sometimes are more clueless about what a Traumatic Brain Injury is and how that injury affects not only the patient but family as well. I continue to learn.

Finding support groups for the caregiver of a TBI patient is almost non-existent because, in part, most couples cannot survive without divorce or separation and finding a common place to meet can logistically make it difficult. But there is hope. There are popular caregiver groups available on the Internet which allow caregivers to share a common grace with each other. And although TBI is different for every patient, the similarities of betrayal and abandonment felt by the spouse can help her/him feel less alienated and alone.

In the first few years after Charlie's wreck, I had no group to help me. However I knew that a therapist for "just me," would be beneficial, but I had to experience several therapists before I found the one professional who was very knowledgeable with brain trauma, and who would be a tremendous support for me not only as a wife but as a caregiver. The key is finding someone who is educated about TBI. To this day, my therapist's wisdom continues to help me as I journey forward in my own life. As a side note, journaling my thoughts (often) has been a necessity for me, especially during sleepless nights. It helps me to better digest every obstacle that confronts me. A valuable tool indeed!

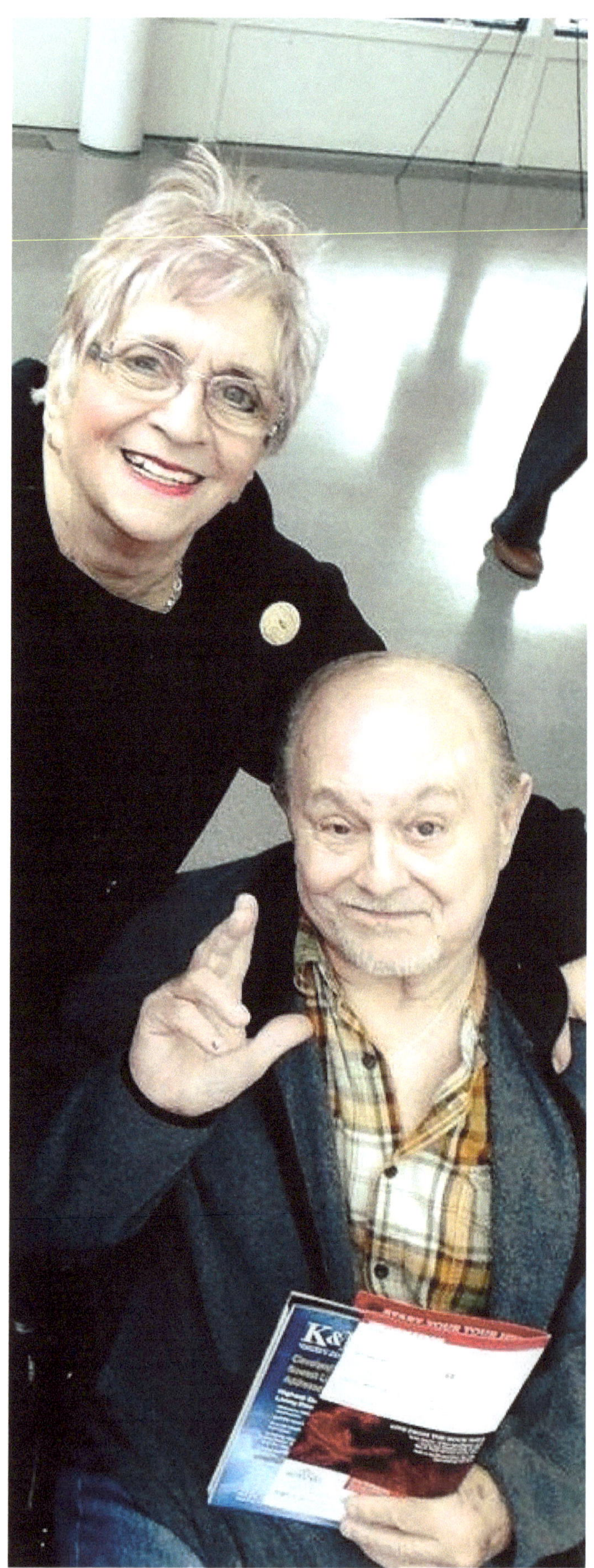

It has now been a long time since some of the best parts of Charlie were destroyed on a highway somewhere in Oklahoma. We both have sacrificed much and worked hard to get to where we are today, but it still hurts. For me, the heartbreak of our earlier memories continues to tear me into small pieces, but not as often anymore. I grieve that which was lost! Yet, I am fortunate because he is able to live at home with me, and is not tethered to a bed or a wheelchair. His memory and confusion continue to plague him, and I must continue to learn the harsh reality of watching my own back, instead of depending on him and his love to bolster me. Over the past eight years, I've come to see he still has some level of love and care for me, as I do for him, but the kind of love is different now.

> **I could say I never thought about walking away from this whole caregiver thing, but that would be a lie.**

I could say I never thought about walking away from this whole caregiver thing, but that would be a lie. And although there are some who deemed it safer and healthier to end their marriages (and they were probably right), I think for us, there had already been so many years invested in the lovely side of love, that staying together is the only option we could choose. For us, it was a right choice.

TBI is a hard and lonely experience to go through, filled with disappointments and uphill battles, but sometimes in life, the most painful lessons are best remembered. Although June will not come back ever as I once thought it would, it has become necessary for me to gather up some of the wise attributes that the month has to offer. June demonstrates a "coming out," from within the center of the darkest winter, and carries upon its arm only the freshest fragrance and most colorful blooms over any other time of the year. With that in mind, I will try to become more like June in my own life. In the end, Charlie and I will carry on together, knowing we didn't really miss June at all! We were simply caught unaware it had arrived!

Meet Barbara Weekley

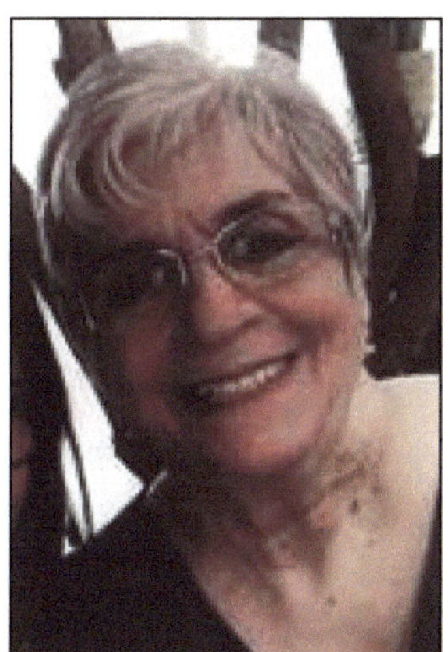

Barbara and her husband Charlie live in northern Ohio in a small community on the shore of Lake Erie. Barbara has been the primary caregiver to her husband in the eight years since his accident.

In 2013, Barbara published a book about her caregiver experience. Barbara's book, "Upright on Broken Limbs," has let her share her caregiver experience with others so they know that they are not alone in their struggles and challenges.

Call Today & Pay Less!
855-605-0234

Digital Starter & Performance Internet

- ✔ 140+ Channels
- ✔ Up to 25 Mbps

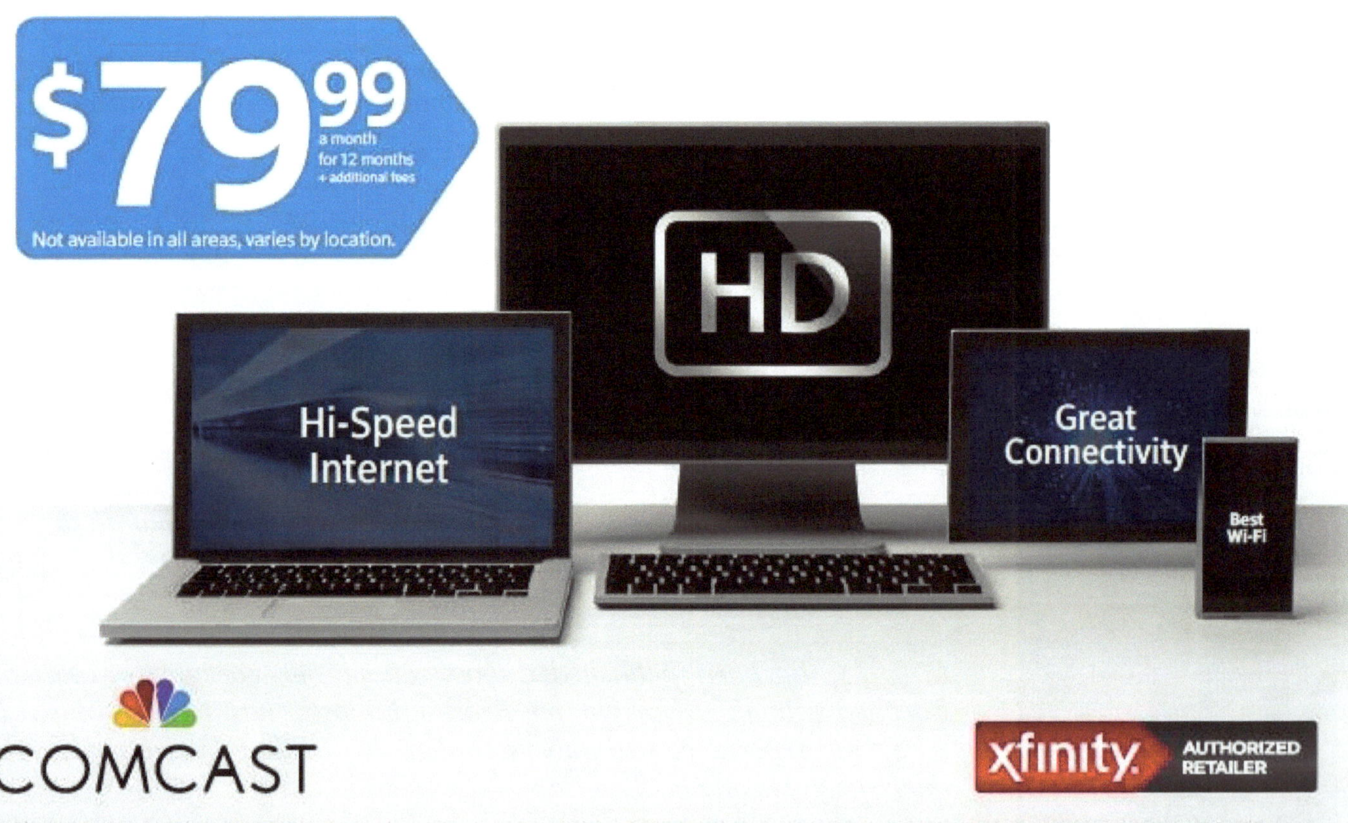

COMCAST

xfinity. AUTHORIZED RETAILER

"""

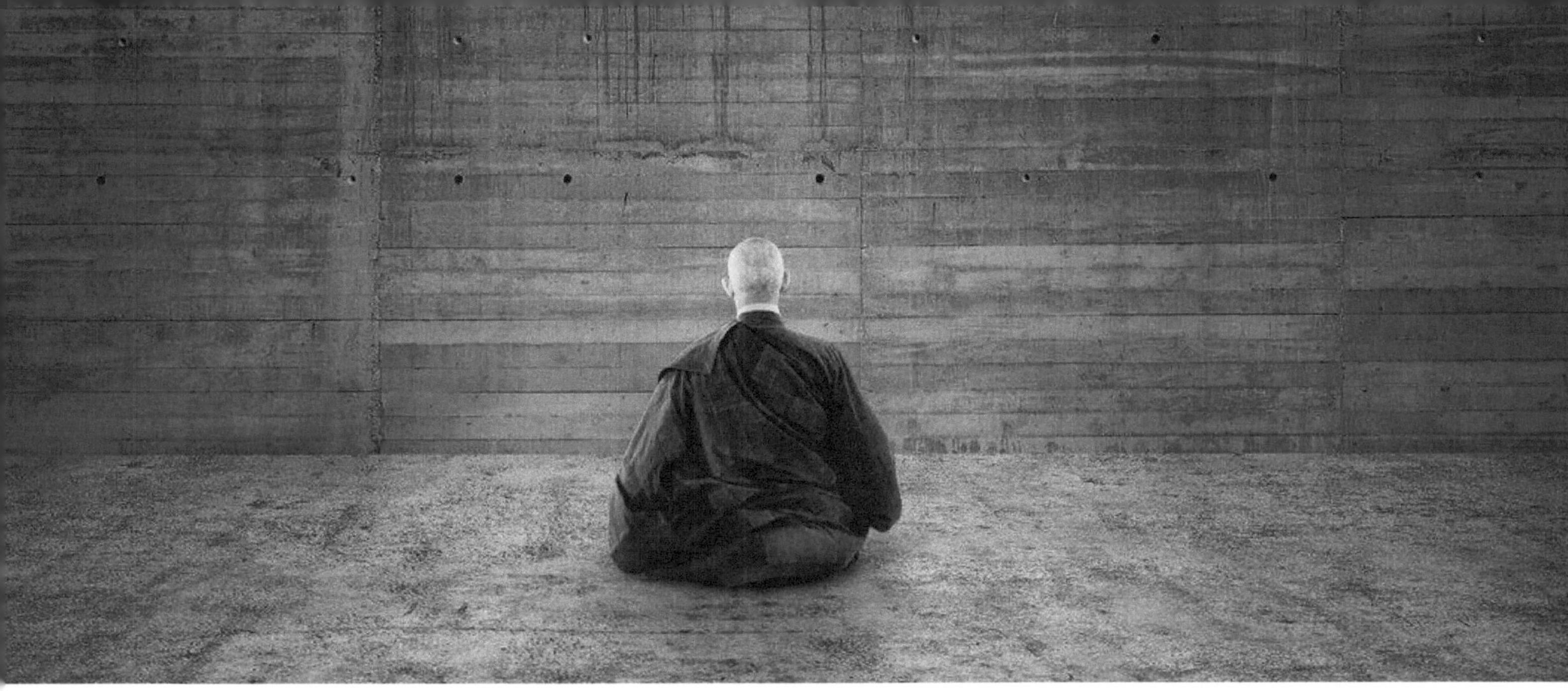

Crash Monty's Laments and Rebirth

By Sean Montgomery

My life changed on March 3, 2015, at 2:45 PM, when I went from being a hard-working treatment technician at Foothills Treatment Plant, helping to produce potable water and megawatts of hydroelectric power for the Denver metropolitan area, to becoming a broken marionette falling twenty feet down into a cistern. I became "Crash Monty," a TBI survivor, spending the last 21 months in rehabilitation!

To be clear, I don't remember the accident or hospital treatment. These details are taken from my wife's journal. In movies, all the details are shown, like who did what, why, and how, but in my case, I don't remember them.

According to the journal, one of my co-workers, Steve, climbed down in the cistern to help me. He probably saved my life, and a lot of my brain function, because I was not breathing when he reached me. He opened my airway until the Flight for Life medics could retrieve me, assess me, and stabilize me as best they could and medevac me to St. Anthony's trauma ward.

What followed was three weeks of coma, strung out on Dilantin and heavy opioid painkillers to keep me sedated and seizure-free. My first memory is from about a month after the accident when Deb, my wife, played lots of jazz, samba, and other happy tunes, reminding me of the joyous dancing adventures of our decade

To be clear, I don't remember the accident or hospital treatment. These details are taken from my wife's journal.

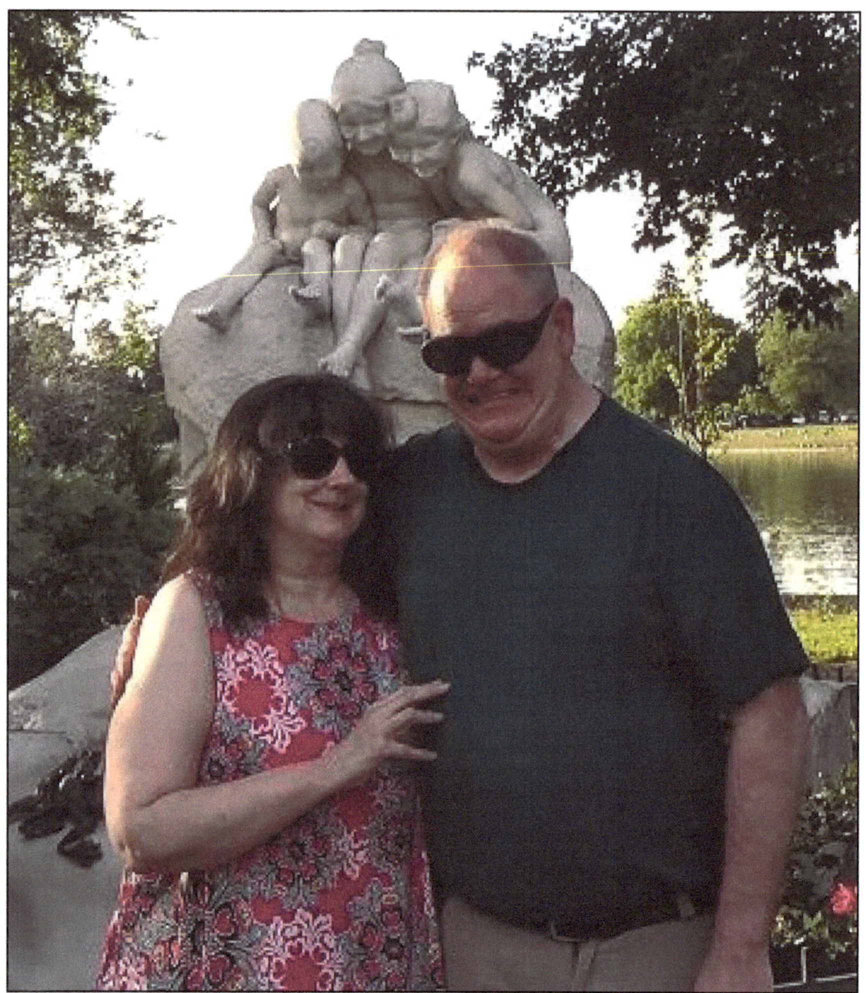

together. When I saw pictures of myself at St. Anthony's, and after Deb informed of the specifics in her journal, I realized how seriously I was injured. Every rib on my left side had been broken. I had liver, spleen, and kidney injuries. I also clipped my collarbone so close to my spine I could very easily have been paralyzed. My left eye socket was smashed, and superior left molars and bicuspids busted. But the worst injuries were to my brain!

I used to be multilingual in five languages besides English: Spanish, German, Russian, Japanese, and Farsi were mastered to college level fluency and literacy. I read vociferously, wrote daily, and remembered lots of what I encountered. However, effects of the fall's multiple bilateral subdural, epidural, and parenchymal hematomas shut all that down. My brain was a bloody, swelling sponge. The fall trashed the intricately interwoven, interdependent network of memory, executive functions, and intuitive "inspirational" insights from my background to sudden, unexpected, but welcome epiphanies. The ironic truth is, as frustrated as I was before my accident with not getting the pay, respect, and responsibilities I deserved as a water treatment professional, I really miss working at Foothills, the sense of being part of a team, and protecting the public's health and welfare.

The one aspect of myself I'd assiduously cultivated and was proud of was my intellect, which was compromised by the injury. My memory, executive mental functions, and wit were not only my shield, goggles for reality, but also my favorite tools. I feel bereft of my magic, strength, and wisdom. I've missed the sense of masculine competence I felt while getting greasy and sweaty on the twelve-hour shifts at Foothills. Yet, the stuff I do now like cooking, housekeeping, and restocking as a volunteer at Metro Caring food bank, isn't bad for somebody "recovering" from being critically injured.

I went from being bedbound to walking on my own less than a year after my fall. I've had to become more patient, better organized, and much easier to satisfy, taking solace in what I CAN do. I have to listen to others' feedback and deal with reality simply as it is, without being lost in my own fantasies to suit my wounded ego!

The simplest and most essential revelation I've gotten from the fall is that every day is a gift, enjoy it as it comes, make what plans I can for success, but not be in any hurry. Prioritize, organize, and see, listen, and feel reality as it is, neutral, harshly impersonal, unjust, and a great challenge.

I rely on my inner Zen monk to be as flexible, adaptable, and resourceful as I can without being a slave to egotism, materialism, and with unmet emotional needs. Today, I don't let my ego tempt me with wild fantasies of unlimited powers and opportunities taking the shorter unethical path. I have to repeat my mantra: "No drama needed or wanted here today!" to keep doing what works. My ego is an irrelevant voice of distraction. The simplest truth is to admit that I'm just a human being with mortal flaws. I have to enjoy the wild gifts of consciousness, an active conscience, and proper senses of humor and humility.

Meet Sean Montgomery

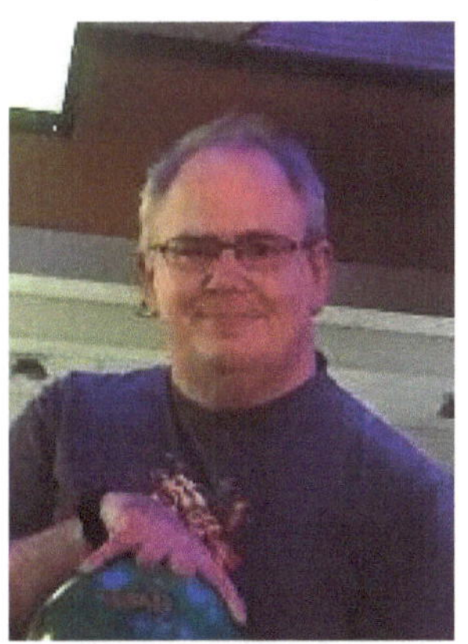

Sean has worked on rehabilitating himself after surviving a 20' fall at work in 2015. As an adult, he has dedicated himself to public service, serving four years' active duty in the US Navy, then eighteen years of work in water treatment. Sean earned his degree in May 2012 at University of Texas in San Antonio.

He is happily married to Deborah Becker and is multilingual in English, Spanish, German, Russian, Japanese, Farsi and Armenian. He also enjoys dancing salsa, jogging, martial arts and reading about anthropology.

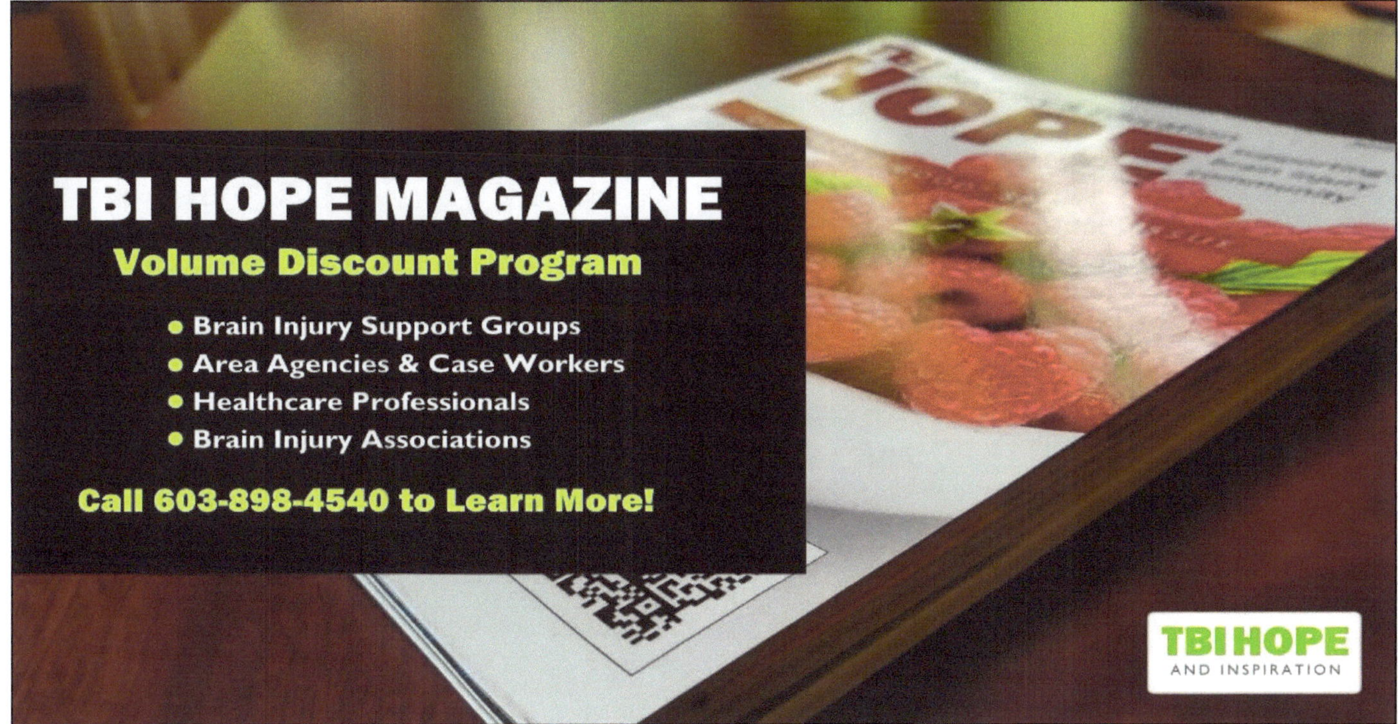

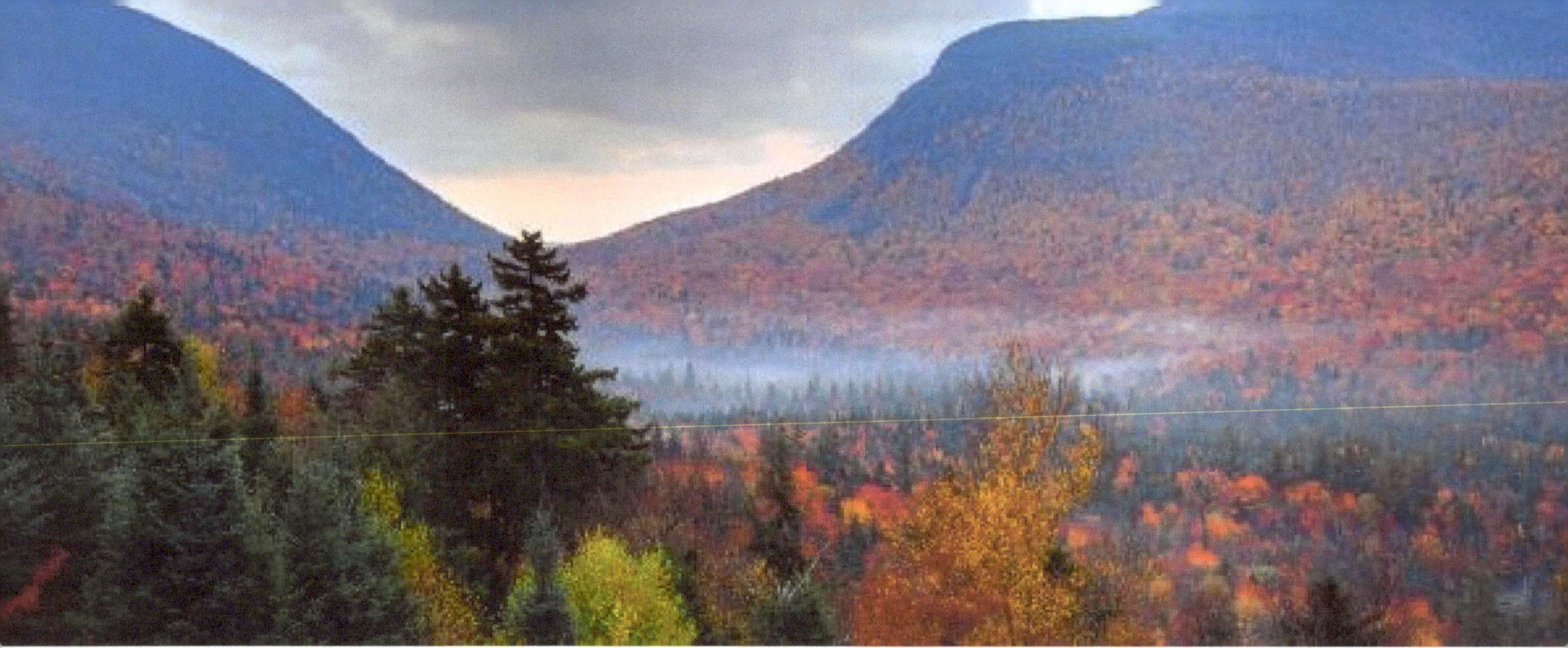

A Day I'll Never Forget

By Angela Nicholson

July 27th is a day that I will never forget. It started out as a normal day. It was the day after my son's ninth birthday, and our family was visiting. We went to dinner after my husband John left for work. Later, we returned home to take our usual family photos by the lilac tree. That's when the call came in, the call that changed everything. I will never forget that call.

"There's been an accident," said the voice on the phone. "John is being brought to the hospital. He has multiple injuries." At that time, I didn't know that the injuries we faced were not minor, but major traumatic injuries, including a traumatic brain injury. I remember rushing to get to him, all while being kept informed of his condition, but no one telling me upfront what was really wrong. When they said he was being life-flighted to Boston, I then knew that this was very serious.

I remember crying in the back seat of the car as my brother-in-law drove me to Boston. I just wanted to see him. By the time I got to the hospital, they had already knocked him out to get him into the helicopter. I remembered thinking, "When will he wake up? When can I talk to him? When will I see him again?" Little did I know, those questions were minor compared to what I was about to face.

John's trauma was very serious. He had injuries to his head, skull, shoulder, leg, arm, eye, and abdomen. Many surgeries awaited him, as well as months of therapy, rehab, and a whole new life.

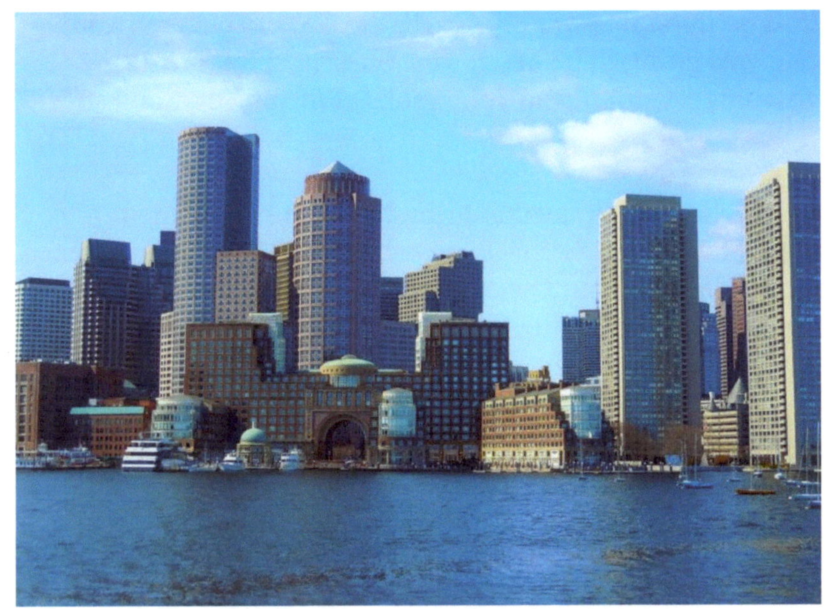

I was stuck in Boston with two young children in an unfamiliar hotel room. Looking back, I don't remember a lot of that time. Some memories are a blur, and some are stuck. The fourteen-hour surgery, the day after he fell, wanting to know that he was okay, waiting to know what they found, and what their thoughts were. Most of those memories are gone.

It was one of the longest days of my life. I remember the doctors saying, "We don't know what he will have when he wakes up. We don't know if he has lost vision in the eye. We won't know the extent of his brain injury until later."

Brain injury. It stuck in my head like a sledgehammer. Would he remember me? Would he remember his kids? Would he know my name, my face? So many things started to run through my mind. I couldn't fathom the fact that there was the possibility of him waking up and not remembering me. I can still see the hospital rooms, the people I talked with, the pacing of the floors, the bench where I sat, calling with updates to family and friends, the hotel I stayed in - the one that became our home away from home.

I can hear the sound of the busy Boston life, the noise, the hustle, and bustle. I can feel the soreness that my feet felt from walking numerous steps in flip flops, the only thing I had to wear. Those things never leave your mind. The day he finally awoke and knew me, but not himself, and the things he didn't know after waking up. Some things I will never forget.

Onto rehab we went, a whole new realm of memories and instances that one never forgets. That year, 2010, was a rough one. No one could have prepared me for the things that were about to change in my life, nor could they have prepared me for how much this would impact me forever. Little things, even. We had numerous appointments in Boston for a year. Every time we made the drive, I had the same chills looking at the same things. It brought back all those memories. The food court on the corner, below where our hotel room was, where my children ate for two weeks. The streets that I knew I had walked numerous times to be with John or to check on the kids; the buildings that we visited in the months following to track progress or have more surgeries. It all was so surreal in the following months. Even now, years later, it's still surreal.

Fast-forward five years to July 27th, 2016. It was the same as the day in 2010, except John has not returned to work. He is permanently disabled, but something isn't right. We both dread this day, whether we talk about it or not. We know it's the anniversary of our new life, the anniversary that brought me a whole new man.

John wasn't feeling well, so I decided to take him to the hospital. Family visiting, like before, so many things the same. They brought John back to the emergency room, and I quickly followed, as they had already done tests and were awaiting a doctor to come in. He kept saying he was sorry, and then it happened. At 7:27 PM, the exact time the call came in on that night in 2010, the doctors came in and informed us that John had had a heart attack. He was going to be taken to another hospital for further testing. Deja vu. So many things were going through my mind, and John looks at me as I cry, and says "Happy Anniversary, I am so sorry."

To this day, I can't get out of my head even the smallest of things that bring back the largest memories. Our family has gone through so much and like most who deal with TBI, we continue to face battles each and every day. I am now a primary caregiver to my husband, and as many memories as I hold in my heart through all that we have endured, the largest memory that tugs at me the strongest is the memory of what was.

Meet Angela Nicholson

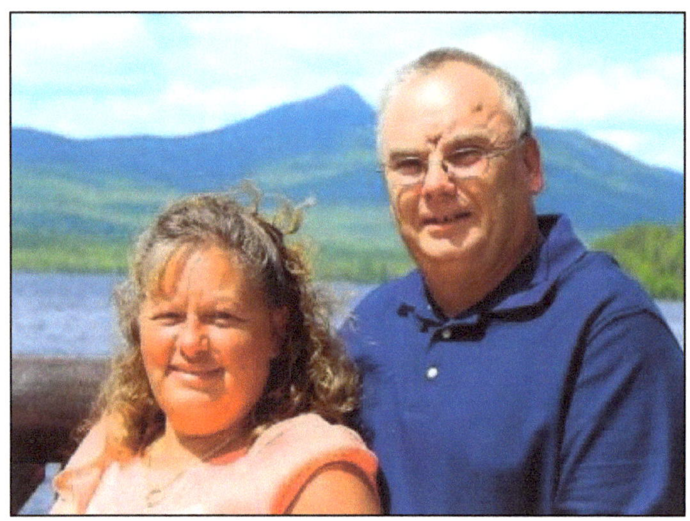

Angela Nicholson is a resident of central New Hampshire after moving there eighteen years ago from Ohio. She has three children, a grandson, and has been married to her husband John for thirteen years. She is a caregiver to her husband, but in her free time she enjoys travelling, spending time with her kids, boating, the ocean, the lakes, watching her son race, and enjoying being a Mimi.

A warm hello to our regular monthly readers at Community Crossroads in Atkinson, NH. We ♥ you guys!

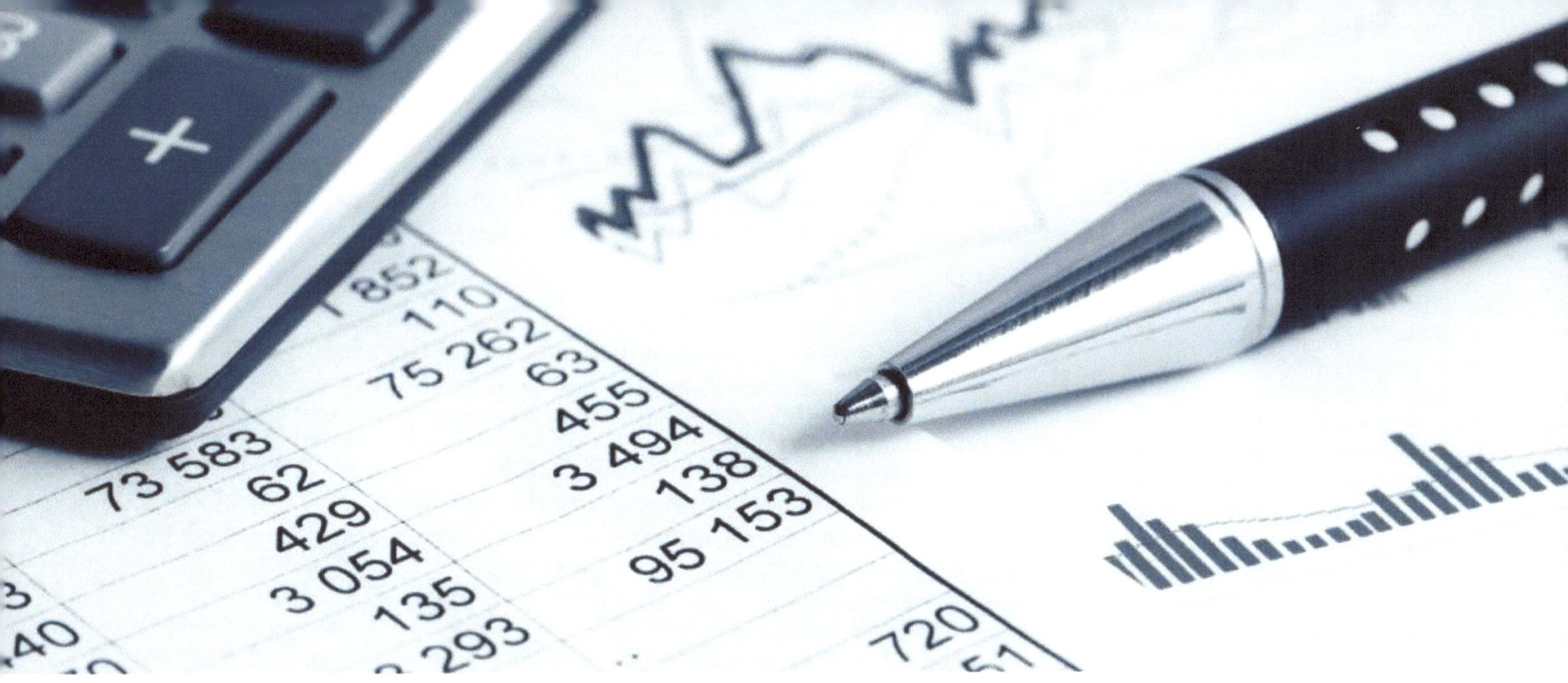

Runaway Spending After Brain Injury

By Thomas Henson Jr. and Carol Svec

The call from my sister started pleasant enough: "Could you send me an early birthday gift?" Ann's voice sounded light, almost happy.

"Sure," I said. "What would you like?"

There was an ominous pause. "What can you afford?"

That was how our family learned about my sister's brain injury finances which spelled financial disaster. Within days we were all sucked in, fighting to rebuild yet another aspect of her life.

> ## We learned that Ann had maxed out seven credit cards. Collection agencies were hounding her.

Ann's brain injury was caused by a fist-sized meningioma and the surgery to remove it. She seemed to thrive until she got divorced five years ago. Then—on her own for the first time—Ann struggled to take over paying household bills. It wasn't until the "birthday present" call that our family learned that this particular task was beyond her capabilities.

We learned that Ann had maxed out seven credit cards. Collection agencies were hounding her. And scammers loved her—she gave the equivalent of six mortgage payments to a "matchmaker" who advertised with a homemade sign on the side of a highway.

Financially, Ann had fallen as far as someone can go without ending up homeless (although she was on her way there, too). My family has become painfully aware of a sad truth: Ann's brain injury took away her "money sense." Managing her finances was simply beyond her ability due to her brain injury.

> **People with brain injury often feel embarrassed and frustrated about the abilities that were stolen from them.**

Runaway spending and inability to manage money are common among people with certain types of brain injury, especially with frontal lobe damage. That's where the "executive functions" reside, including the abilities to plan, make decisions, process information, and control inappropriate behavior, such as spending a year's salary on shoes or football tickets. These changes can be called "brain injury finances."

Despite the sometimes staggering levels of debt, families often don't see the problem. Unlike other behaviors, spending is almost magical—wave a plastic card, and "poof!" you're now $20,000 deeper in debt. It's quick and invisible (unless shopping bags start piling up). Plus, in many families, money is a taboo topic. But that attitude only fosters silence, secrets, and shame, followed by emergency calls begging for help.

Here are solutions to these brain injury finances that we have found helpful, some with specific notes for families and individuals with brain injury:

Open a dialog, and open the books.

People with brain injury often feel embarrassed and frustrated about the abilities that were stolen from them. This can make it difficult to admit to yet another area of disability.

Families: You'll get more straight answers if you create an atmosphere of acceptance that is free of blame.

Individual: The conversation will be difficult, but stick with it. Be honest. Only then can you put together a workable plan for getting you out of debt.

Define the problem.

With investigation, patterns will emerge. Is the problem one of spending too much? Not writing checks in a timely manner? Poor record-keeping? From that understanding you can put processes in place to address the issues.

Get the family involved.

Families: The problem of unfettered spending may require constant supervision. Consider appointing a family member to take over the checkbook and do monthly reviews of finances.

Individuals: As difficult as it may be to relinquish control, the solution to your financial worries may require more hands-on help from your family. It may help to think of it as allowing your family to take over the stress of money.

Sign up for notifications.

Banks and credit card companies can provide email notifications when bank account funds dip below a specified level, or when spending increases above a certain dollar amount. Sign up for these notifications so that there are no major surprises from month to month.

Assign a Limited Power of Attorney.

Power of Attorney (POA) allows a specified family member to have access to an individual's accounts and financial records so they can monitor spending and perform other financial activities.

Finally, understand that you don't have to go it alone. There are experts who can help. Ask your doctor or attorney for referrals to reputable experts who may be useful. For example, *Life Care Planners* provide guidance for the "big picture." They can help assess current and future financial needs—throughout your entire lifetime—and formulate a plan to best maintain your quality of life. *Case Managers* deal with the nuts and bolts of daily living, such as learning how to set up procedures for remembering to pay bills, or arranging for transportation if necessary. And if the situation is truly dire, consider talking with a bankruptcy attorney.

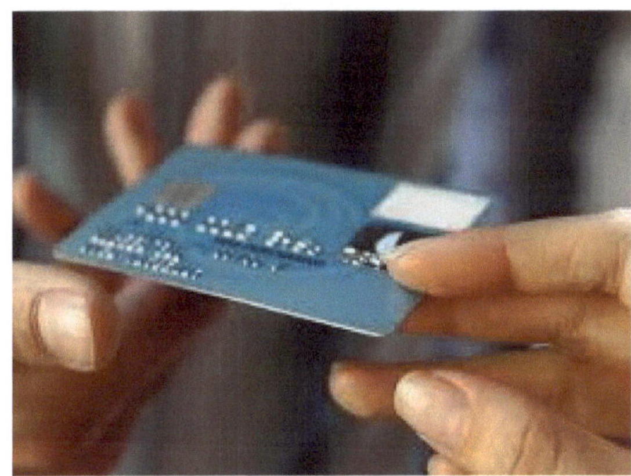

Under the best of circumstances, money problems are difficult, and brain injury compounds the strain. As you struggle to climb out of the financial trenches, keep family close - as a resource and as support. It's easier to climb up when you have strong shoulders to stand on.

Meet the Authors

Thomas Henson Jr. is a partner and Head of the Complex Litigation Group at HensonFuerst Attorneys, based in Raleigh and Rocky Mount, NC. He serves on the board of directors of the Brain Injury Association of North Carolina (BIANC), and in 2012, Thomas was appointed by the governor to a four-year term on the North Carolina Traumatic Brain Injury Advisory Council.

Thomas remains an active member of the Traumatic Brain Injury Litigation Group of the American Association for Justice.

Carol Svec is the creative director at HensonFuerst Attorneys, and an award-winning health and wellness writer. She is also a loving sister to Ann, whose story was told in this article.

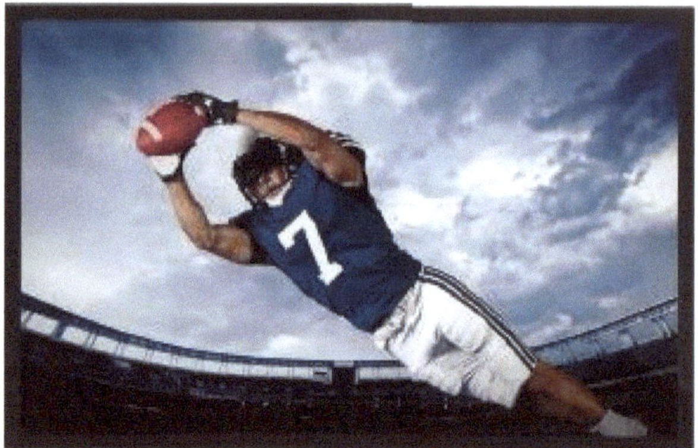

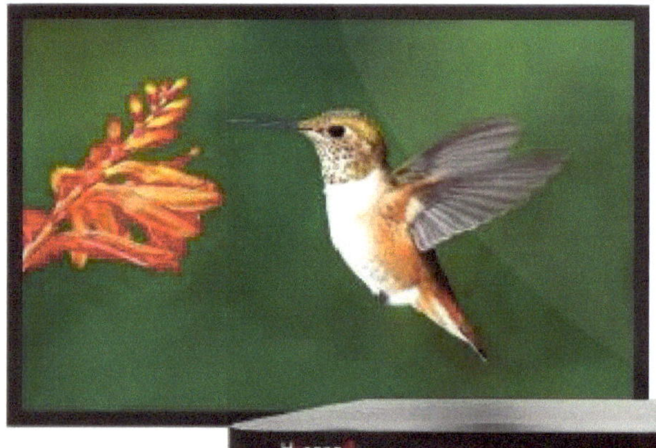

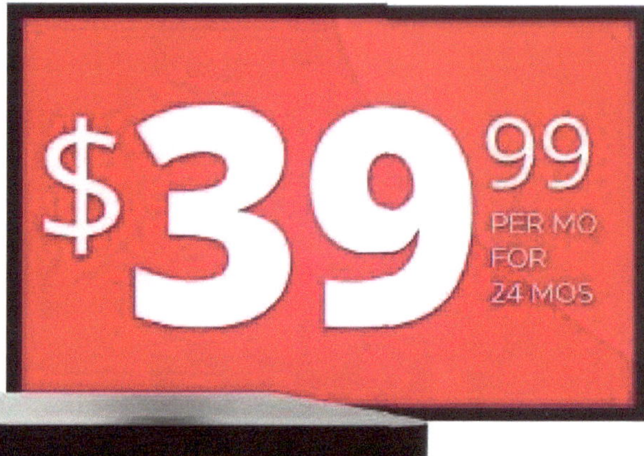

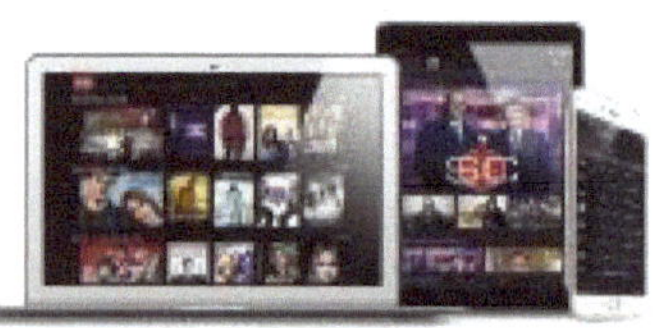

+

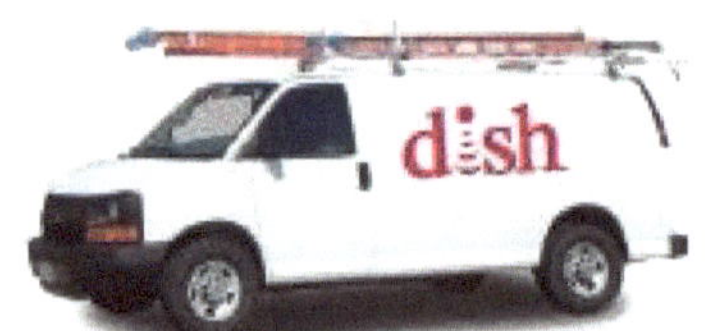

+

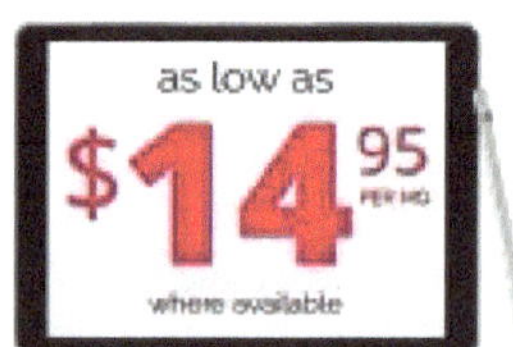

Call 1-800-391-1328

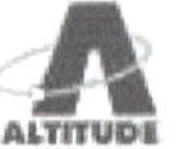

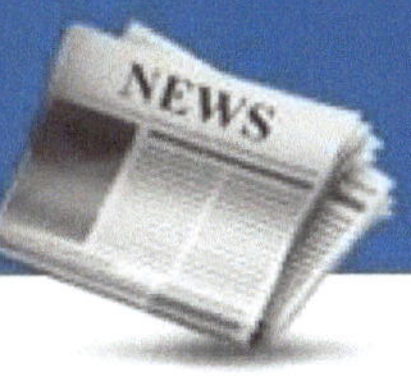

If you've made it this far, you've just completed reading the thirty-first issue of TBI HOPE Magazine. We marvel that the three year anniversary of our publication's launch is approaching. Our magazine is now read monthly in over forty countries around the globe. We have readers on every continent except Antarctica. It's hard not to be both humbled and amazed by the growth of our magazine.

It has become increasingly clear that survivors, family members as well as members of the medical and professional community have an unmet need to hear survivor's stories *as told in their own voices*. We are grateful to be a catalyst for this, helping others to learn and better understand what brain injury families live with.

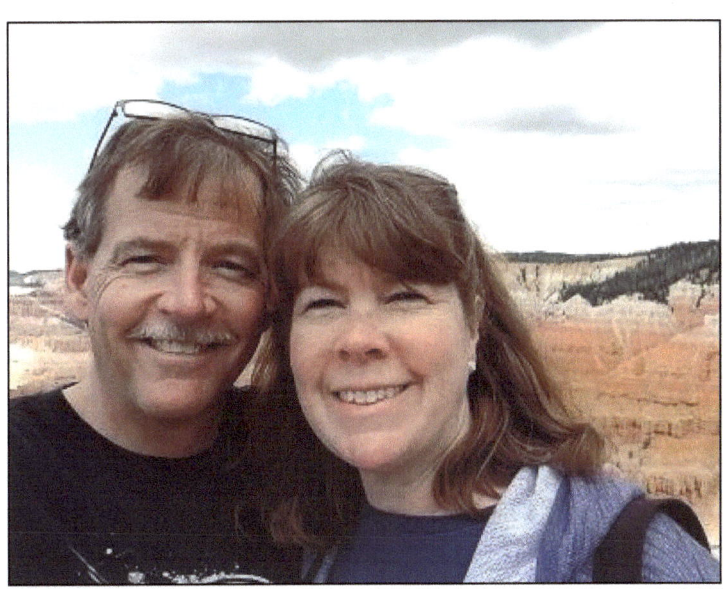

This past week, we received a deeply moving email. Members of a local support group penned short notes about what TBI HOPE Magazine has meant to them. The email moved Sarah and I more deeply than most will ever know or understand. As members of a survivor family, we understand the day-to-day challenges so many others face.

Though it has been shared a few times since we launched the print version of TBI HOPE Magazine earlier this year, it is worth sharing again – we offer qualifying organizations a very deep discount on the print version of our publication. For years, readers asked for the publication in print, something we are profoundly grateful to offer now.

To those regular readers who take the time to reach out to us, you already know that every email gets a reply. If you have something that you think will better our publication, don't be shy. And for those who have already reached out to us with comments and suggestions, thank you!

Peace to all with lives affected by brain injury,

~David & Sarah